AIDS

A Strategy for Nursing Care

Robert J. Pratt

RN, BA, MSc, RGN, RNT, DipN (Lond)

Vice Principal (Faculty of Continuing Education)
Riverside College of Nursing
London

Third Edition

Edward Arnold
A division of Hodder & Stoughton
LONDON   MELBOURNE   AUCKLAND

© 1991 Robert J. Pratt

First published in Great Britain 1986
Third impression 1987
Second Edition 1988
Third impression 1989
AISE edition first published in 1988
Third edition 1991

British Library Cataloguing in Publication Data
Pratt, Robert J.
    AIDS : a strategy for nursing care.—Rev. ed.
    1. AIDS patients. Care
    I. Title
    362.1969792

    ISBN 0–340–54841–X

Whilst the advice and information in this book are believed to be
true and accurate at the date of going to press, neither the author nor
the publisher can accept any legal responsibility or liability for any
errors or omissions that may be made.

Printed and bound in Great Britain for Edward Arnold a division of
Hodder and Stoughton Limited, Mill Road, Dunton Green,
Sevenoaks, Kent TN13 2YA by Biddles Ltd., Guildford and
King's Lynn.

Contents

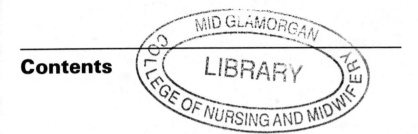

Foreword

We are now entering the second decade of our experience of caring for individuals with AIDS and HIV-related health problems. In the United Kingdom, the Riverside Health Authority is at the very epicentre of this global pandemic and as such, we are caring for large numbers of individuals who are unwell as a result of HIV infection. Although our knowledge of the underlying science and pathology driving this epidemic has increased, there still has not emerged a biomedical 'cure' for this disease. The need for nurses to 'care' is as urgent now as when the disease first surfaced.

The first two editions of this important book established a knowledge base for nurses seeking a technical, managerial, professional and ethical strategy for caring for an ever increasing number of frightened young men and women infected with HIV. In this third edition, the author seeks to not only update the previous information, but also to move the reader on to consider the wider issues involved in directing this strategy towards the creation of a more 'HIV aware' health care organisation. In this book, the author shares with you an attempt to create an ethical framework to ensure that we offer all our clients the highest possible quality of care. This edition incorporates both technical and professional standards of care which have evolved within the Riverside Health Authority and which now form the basis of a model for nursing and for professional decision making.

The numbers of individuals infected with human immunodeficiency viruses (HIV) will continue to increase for many years to come. Although AIDS and HIV infection has not produced any new professional issues, it has highlighted the need to re-explore our professional responses when confronted with people who have a right to expect confident, competent and compassionate care.

The author has made a major national and local contribution in facilitating the nursing profession's early, effective response to the challenges of AIDS in the United Kingdom.

I would urge you not only to use this book as the definitive textbook on the nursing care of individuals with AIDS and HIV-related conditions that it is, but to allow the issues that it raises to stimulate you to question and define your professional and clinical practice.

Chris Beasley
Chief Nurse Adviser to the Riverside Health Authority, Nurse Representative to the UK Department of Health's *Expert Advisory Group on AIDS* (EAGA)

1991

I am indebted to Evangeline A. Karn, Head of the Department for Clinical Studies in the Riverside College of Nursing, for her patient proof-reading and advice on style. I am also grateful to the course members of ENB Course No. 934 (The Care and Management of Individuals with AIDS and HIV-related Conditions) at the Riverside College of Nursing, for their new insights into the nursing management of individuals with HIV-related conditions.

This text is dedicated to the patients and nursing staff of the Riverside Health Authority, London.

Robert Pratt
1991

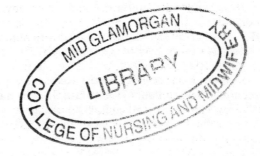

Introduction

> In the face of intense and immediate crisis, when an outbreak of
> plague implanted fear of imminent death in an entire community,
> ordinary routines and customary restraints broke down. Rituals
> arose to discharge anxiety and local panic often provoked bizarre
> behavior. The first efforts at ritualizing responses to the plague took
> extreme and ugly forms.
> *Plagues and Peoples*. W.H. McNeill.

Shortly before Christmas in 1981, the first patient with AIDS in the
United Kingdom lay dying in a London hospital. Medical and nursing
experts, casting a nervous glance at the United States where over three
hundred cases of this new disease had been identified, probably knew
from the beginning that the UK would not escape this developing
epidemic.

As 1982 and 1983 came and went, more cases were seen and, in a
sense, our worst fears were realized. Cases of AIDS were no longer
being imported into the UK but rather, we had our own endemic brand,
which was quickly spreading. Certain aspects of this particular disease
were especially alarming; its cause was unknown as was its means of
spread. Treatment of the various infections and cancers seen in this disease was ineffective, no-one surviving once the disease took hold.
Almost all of the affected were young adults, mostly men, and fear of
the disease became a parallel epidemic in its own right.

The heady months of 1984 brought both good news and bad news.
Brilliant research work by French scientists the year before had
uncovered the causative agent of AIDS. This was now confirmed by
researchers in America. With this discovery, the different ways in which
the epidemic was spreading also became clear and it seemed only a
matter of time before a vaccine would be available to stop, once and for
all, this ferocious disease. Nurses, however, noticed that increasing
numbers of patients, either with AIDS or under investigation for AIDS-
related conditions, continued to be admitted, and, thanks to the
hysteria and panic whipped up by a sensation-seeking media, health
care workers became as confused and frightened as everyone else. As

always, the twenty-four hour care of these patients, like all other patients, was the paramount responsibility of nurses and they often seemed surrounded by frightened and sometimes hostile ancillary staff; domestics refusing to clean patients' rooms, catering staff refusing to serve meal trays to patients with AIDS, porters refusing to transport patients with this disease and undertakers refusing to accept the bodies of patients who had died from AIDS. Even some medical staff, (notably surgeons), would refuse to treat patients who had AIDS. Draconian infectious disease control procedures, bearing no logical relationship to the known facts of transmission, were often implemented, regardless of cost either in nursing time or in the further, deepening sense of isolation of these patients, frightened of becoming ever more abandoned.

In 1985, 165 new cases brought the total number of individuals in the UK with AIDS to 273. The Communicable Disease Surveillance Centre suggested that as the numbers continued to increase, in 1988, 2000 new cases might reasonably be expected[1].

This year (1985) also saw the introduction of a blood test which could detect previous exposure to the AIDS virus. This test showed that not all individuals infected with the AIDS virus went on to develop AIDS; others developed a less severe illness as a consequence of infection. Many remained healthy, free of any clinical symptoms, but *infected and infectious*. The Chief Medical Officer for the Department of Health and Social Security estimated that there might be over 10 000 such individuals in the UK (estimates of asymptomatic infected individuals in the USA ranged from 500 000 to one and a half million)[2]. Not only were these large numbers of infected individuals now able to escalate the epidemic dramatically, but also suspicion grew that these thousands of asymptomatic carriers might not remain asymptomatic as the years went by. It was known by 1985 that the AIDS virus not only attacked the immune system, but also attacked cells in the brain, leading, in many cases, to dementia[3]. It seemed reasonable to speculate that everyone infected with this virus would eventually suffer some form of ill health as a consequence. No health care system, in any part of the world, including the National Health Service in the UK, seemed prepared for even the present number of cases of people with fully expressed AIDS. How they would cope with the 'worst case' scenario of caring for increased numbers of currently asymptomatic infected individuals was not a pleasant thought to contemplate.

By 1986, there was not the least doubt that AIDS and AIDS-related conditions posed the most significant public health issue of our time. Not only were there the American and European epidemics, but major epidemics were also occurring in Central Africa, South America and in Australia. AIDS had become of truly pandemic proportions. It was clear that it would be with us, in our hospitals and in our communities for years to come.

By the end of 1988 over 2000 individuals in the UK had been diagnosed as having fully-expressed AIDS and for each individual with AIDS there were 5–10 individuals with lesser forms of ill-health as a direct consequence of infection. By December, 1988 it was estimated that there may have been as many as 26 400 individuals in the United Kingdom infected with the virus which can cause AIDS and that by the end of 1990, this number would increase in England and Wales to 46 450. By early 1990, over 3 000 individuals in the United Kingdom had been diagnosed as having AIDS and this number was likely to grow to 10 600 in England and Wales by the end of 1993[4]. Both Scotland and Northern Ireland were also seeing an accelerated growth in the epidemic.

Dealing with the disease one day at a time, and one patient at a time, professional nurses have built up considerable expertise in developing individualized nursing care strategies, designed to deliver compassionate, non-judgemental, efficient and effective nursing care to large numbers of relatively young people, suffering and dying in fear and confusion. It is the nurse who cares for these patients. This text has been written to provide guidance and support, to share collective expertise, to reassure and to inform. Like our predecessors in the great epidemics of the past, nurses must be brave in the face of this current epidemic. We cannot abandon any of our patients, nor would we wish to do so. With accurate information, planned nursing care can be designed to safely and competently meet the needs of patients suffering from one of the most devastating diseases seen in recent times. On the eve of World War II, the American President, Franklin D. Roosevelt, told the American people, '. . . we have nothing to fear except fear itself'. For health care workers confronting the calamity of AIDS in the 1990s, the same is equally true. The enemy is not only the AIDS virus, but equally, fear, ignorance and prejudice. If in a small way this text neutralizes some of these factors, it will have been worth the effort.

References

1. Acheson, E.D. (1985). The CMO's briefing on AIDS. *THS Health Summary*. 2(VIII) August, pp 6–7
2. Acheson, E.D. (1986). AIDS: A challenge for the public health. *Lancet*. i(8482), March 22, pp 662–6
3. Sattaur, O. More evidence for brain disease in AIDS. *New Scientist*. 10 October 1985, p 26
4. PHLS Communicable Disease Surveillance Centre (1990). Acquired Immune Deficiency Syndrome in England and Wales to End of 1993 – Projections using data to end September 1989: Report of a Working Group ('The Day Report'), *Communicable Disease Report* (January), UK

1

The Evolving Epidemic

The Plague had swallowed up everything and everyone. No longer were there individual destinies, only a collective destiny, made of plague and the emotions shared by all. Strongest of these emotions was the sense of exile and of deprivation, with all the cross-currents of revolt and fear set up by these.

The Plague. Albert Camus

In the early months of 1981, five young men were admitted to various hospitals in Los Angeles, suffering from an unusual type of pneumonia caused by a commonly occurring protozoa known as *Pneumocystis carinii*. Previously, pneumonia caused by *P. carinii* had only been seen in patients who were immunocompromised, such as infants born with a primary immune deficiency (e.g. severe combined immune deficiency – 'SCID') or in adults whose immune system became deficient due to other causes, i.e. secondary immune deficiency states. Most cases of pneumonia caused by *P. carinii* had been observed in renal transplant units where patients had received immunosuppressant chemotherapy following kidney transplants, or in oncology units, where patients had been immunosuppressed as a result of receiving anti-cancer chemotherapy. Most individuals have been exposed to this microbe and it is part of the normal flora of many people. In individuals with a competent immune system it is harmless. Only in individuals with a faulty immune system can it cause disease, in which case the treatment of choice was a little-used antibiotic manufactured in the United Kingdom known as pentamidine isethionate. The physician in charge of the five cases in Los Angeles was puzzled. These five patients were all young men who had evidence of a widespread immunodeficiency without any apparent reason. They had evidence of other infections and, coincidentally, they were all homosexual. The Centers for Disease Control (CDC) in Atlanta, Georgia, was notified and supplies of pentamidine were requested, although by this time, two of the five patients had died. The CDC, which has as part of its function the task of monitoring the trend of infectious diseases throughout the United

States and its territories, published an account of these five cases in its weekly bulletin, the *Morbidity and Mortality Weekly Report* (MMWR) on 5 June, 1981 and noted that the occurrence of pneumonia caused by *P. carinii* ('pneumocystosis') in five previously healthy individuals, who had no known reason for their defective immune status, was unusual, and questioned whether their homosexual lifestyle, or a disease acquired through sexual contact, could be associated with the development of the defects in the immune system which led to pneumocystosis[1].

Probably then no-one actually suspected the magnitude of the epidemic that was in the making. However, evidence of the gathering storm was soon starting to arrive.

At about the same time as physicians in Los Angeles had reported the cluster of cases of pneumocystosis, physicians in New York City and California notified the CDC of the occurrence of a severe form of Kaposi's sarcoma in 26 young men. Kaposi's sarcoma is a vascular neoplasm, uncommon in the United States and in Western Europe, being seen mainly in elderly men where it is manifested by skin lesions and a chronic clinical course (mean survival time is 8–13 years). However, in 1978 Kaposi's sarcoma had been described in patients who had undergone renal transplants and had received immunosuppressant therapy and in others who were iatrogenically immunosuppressed.

Of the 26 patients reported to the CDC in July of 1981, all had evidence of an immunodeficiency not related to any known cause, and several had other serious infections (four having pneumocystosis). All were homosexual[2].

Simultaneously, an additional 10 cases of pneumocystosis in healthy young gay men in Los Angeles and San Francisco were reported, two of whom also had Kaposi's sarcoma. All these patients had evidence of immunodeficiency with no known underlying cause. The following month saw an additional 70 cases of these two conditions[3]. It was then clear that an epidemic was brewing. This was an epidemic in which death would be caused by one or more unusual, opportunistic infections or by cancer, present only because the immune system had broken down due to unknown reasons.

Extremely alarmed, the CDC instituted a nation-wide surveillance programme in July 1981. The new disease was termed the **Acquired Immune Deficiency Syndrome** and it was characterized as the occurrence of unusual infections or cancers in previously healthy individuals, due to an immunodeficiency of unknown cause.

Data coming into the CDC from investigators all over the United States showed that the incidence of AIDS was roughly doubling every six months. In September 1982, more than two cases were being diagnosed every day and by March 1983, an average of 4–5 cases per day

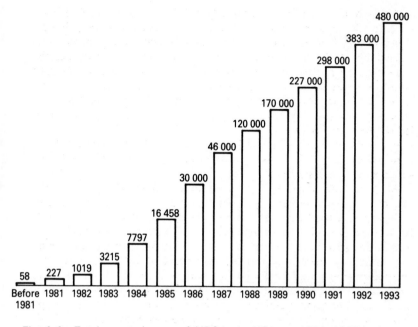

Fig. 1.1 Total reported cases of AIDS in the USA pre-1981–1990 and projected to end of 1993 (adjusted by 18% for under-reporting)

were being reported to the CDC. The total number of cases reported to CDC from prior to 1981 and projected through to the end of 1993 is indicated in Fig. 1.1. Between 1990 and the end of 1993, 480 000 new cases will be reported (98 000 new cases will be diagnosed in 1993 alone) and a total of 340 000 individuals will die of AIDS during this same period.[4]

In addition to cases of fully expressed AIDS, many individuals in the same groups as those 'at risk' of developing fully expressed AIDS (e.g. gay men) were presenting for investigation or treatment with a lesser form of AIDS, which came to be referred to as the AIDS-Related Complex (ARC). Individuals with ARC frequently had a combination of various indicators of ill-health without having frank opportunistic infections or other conditions described in the surveillance definition of AIDS. Frequently they presented with unexplained, persistent and generalized swollen lymph glands (this by itself became known as either 'persistent, generalized lymphadenopathy' – PGL, or the 'lymphadenopathy syndrome' – LAS), almost always including cervical and axillary lymph nodes[5]. In addition, individuals with ARC frequently complained of fever, profuse night sweats, fatigue and weight loss. All

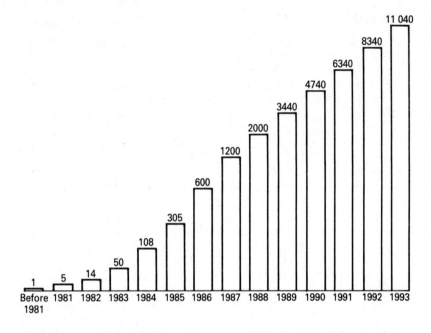

Fig. 1.2   Total reported cases of AIDS in the UK Pre-1981–1990 and projected to end of 1993 (England and Wales only)

these patients showed abnormalities in tests for cell-mediated immunity. Most individuals with ARC progress to fully expressed AIDS. ARC is discussed in detail in Chapter 5.

For every case of AIDS, there would be ten cases of ARC. The numbers started to look astronomical.

Towards the end of 1981, the first patient diagnosed as suffering from AIDS was seen in a London hospital[6] – AIDS had arrived in the United Kingdom.

Data released from the Communicable Disease Surveillance Centre (CDSC) at Colindale reflected a similar pattern of spread to that seen in the United States. Indeed, the growth of new cases reflected the American pattern; it was merely three years behind. The number of UK cases is illustrated in Fig. 1.2. By March 1990, 3021 individuals in the UK had been diagnosed as having AIDS[8] and current projections indicate that this number will increase in England and Wales to a minimum of 11 040 cases by the end of 1993.[7]

Most individuals contracting AIDS are men, and are in the age range 20–49 years, the median age being 34.

'At risk' of infection

Although in both the United States and the United Kingdom AIDS was first recognised in young, male homosexuals, it became clear from the early months of the epidemic that AIDS was not confined to either group. Most individuals in whom AIDS has been diagnosed were men with either homosexual or bisexual life styles. Also at risk were injecting substance misusers, persons with haemophilia, the heterosexual sex partners of persons with AIDS or 'at risk' for AIDS, recipients of transfused blood or blood components, or children from families in which the mother was infected with HIV, the virus which can cause AIDS. Figure 1.3 shows the collated average percentage breakdown of the different groups of individuals who have developed AIDS in the United States and in the United Kingdom.

Although currently most cases of fully expressed AIDS in the UK are seen in gay men, current data indicates that major changes in sexual behaviour in the homosexual community might have been occuring in the mid-1980s. Since this period, evidence has strengthened that transmission of the aetiological agent of AIDS has diminished markedly in gay and bi-sexual men. It is probable that at the end of 1988, somewhere between 8 750 and 17 500 gay and bi-sexual men in England and Wales were infected with HIV. Current projections are that the numbers of new AIDS cases among homosexuals in England and Wales in 1993 are

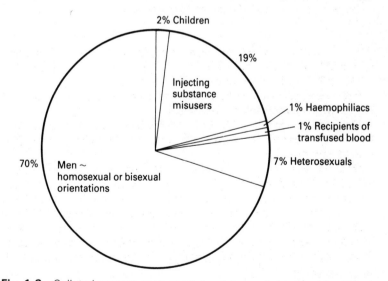

Fig. 1.3 Collated average percentage breakdown of groups of individuals who have developed AIDS in the USA and UK

in the range of 875 to 1500, from a total of 2700 new cases which will be reported in that year alone.[8]

The second major wave of HIV infection and AIDS cases will occur in the injecting substance misuse group and in individuals infected as a result of heterosexual contact. It remains uncertain as to how fast the epidemic will spread through these groups but continuing exponential growth in the number of new persons infected with HIV in both populations is consistent with available data on AIDS diagnoses. If this is so, by 1993, two thirds or more of new AIDS cases and the majority of persons infected with HIV in England and Wales will arise from these two exposure categories.[9]

Groupings of individuals whose behaviour or 'life events' may have predisposed them to risk of HIV infection vary in different parts of the world. In Africa, homosexuals do not make up a significant number of individuals who have AIDS and it is a salutary fact to remember that the vast majority of individuals throughout the world infected with HIV, have become so as a result of heterosexual exposure to this virus. Consequently, as more women become infected, the numbers of children, born infected with the virus which can cause AIDS, will continue to escalate.

AIDS in Europe

The first European cases were seen, it is now realized, before 1979, in France and West Germany and by 30 June 1989, over 24 894 cases throughout Europe had been reported to the World Health Organization Collaborating Centre[10]. AIDS was to be seen in every country in Western Europe and, by 1986, reports of AIDS in Eastern European countries were being published. In general, the same 'at risk' groups were seen in European cases, with one exception. That was the experience in France and Belgium, where there was a relatively high incidence related to the 'African connection'. Many of the cases reported in these two countries were African immigrants from the upper Congo basin or European visitors to that area, principally Zaïre, Uganda, Chad and Ghana.

AIDS – Worldwide

As of 1 September, 1989, the culumative total of AIDS cases reported to the World Health Organisation (WHO) was over 177 000 and WHO estimated the real number to be over 500 000. WHO estimated that 5–6 million people in the World were infected with HIV by mid-1988 and that the total culumative adult AIDS cases throughout the world would reach 5–6 million and the total number of individuals infected with HIV would be over 14 million by the year 2000.[11]

Mortality

Aids is a condition associated with an extremely high case fatality rate. The individual prognosis in people with AIDS varies according to their presenting illnesses. Individuals presenting with opportunistic infections have a poorer prognosis than those who initially present with Kaposi's sarcoma.

In England and Wales, the current (1990) median survival time from date of diagnosis to death is between 18–20 months.[12]

The introduction of zidovudine and other anti-retroviral agents (e.g. dideoxycytidine) and prophylaxis of opportunistic infections in individuals infected with HIV will further increase survival time in the future.

References

1. Centers for Disease Control (1981). Pneumocystis pneumonia. Los Angeles, *Morbidity and Mortality Weekly Report (MMWR)* (June 5), **30**(21):250–2
2. Centers for Disease Control (1981). Kaposi's sarcoma and pneumocystis pneumonia among homosexual men. New York City and California, *MMWR* (July 3), **30**(25):305–8
3. Centers for Disease Control (1981). Follow-up on Kaposi's sarcoma and pneumocystis pneumonia. *MMWR* (August 28), **30**(33):409–10
4. Centers for Disease Control (1990). Current Trends: Estimates of HIV Prevalence and Projected AIDS Cases: Summary of a Workshop October 31-November 1, 1989, *MMWR* (February 22) **39**(7):110–119
5. Centers for Disease Control (1982). Persistent, generalized lymphadenopathy among homosexual males, *MMWR* (May 21), **31**(19):249–51
6. Dubois, R.M., *et al.* (1981). Primary Pneumocystis carinii and cytomegalovirus infection, *Lancet* (December 12) **ii**(8259):1339
7. PHLS Communicable Disease Surveillance Centre (1990). Acquired Immune Deficiency Syndrome in England and Wales to End 1993, Projections Using Data to End September 1989 (Report of a Working Group – Day, N.E., et. al.), *Communicable Disease Report* (January) UK
8. ibid.
9. ibid.
10. Health Education Authority (1990). *AIDS – UK*, Issue 7 (January 1990) UK
11. Sato, P.A., Chin, J., Mann, J.M. (1989). Review of AIDS and HIV infection: global epidemiology and statistics, in *AIDS 1989 A Year in Review*, **3**(Supplement 1):S301–307
12. PHLS Communicable Disease Surveillance Centre (1990). *op. cit.*

2

AIDS – The Cause

From the beginning of the epidemic, AIDS exhibited all the classic signs of an infectious disease and the only convincing explanation for its cause was the emergence of a new infectious agent. An infective aetiology was consistent with the geographical clustering of early cases and epidemiological proof of case-to-case contact[1,2], the newness of the disease, the pattern of groups at risk, its occurrence, within the same time scale, in the diverse groups affected, and finally, its exponential spread. Various researchers independently discovered the causative agent of AIDS at approximately the same time and named the virus responsible: LAV – the lymphadenopathy-associated virus[3], HTLV-III – Human T cell leukemia (lymphotropic) virus type III[4], and ARV– AIDS-associated retrovirus[5]. In May 1986 a subcommittee of the International Committee on the Taxonomy of Viruses proposed that the AIDS retroviruses be officially designated as the 'human immunodeficiency viruses' (HIV).

Characteristics of viruses

All viruses have certain characteristics which distinguish them from other microbes. These characteristics have to do with their composition, shape, method of reproduction, size and their viral antigenic characters and host cell receptors to which they are attracted (Fig. 2.1).

Composition

Genome   The core of the virus is composed of **nucleic acid**. The nucleic acid is *either* DNA (deoxyribonucleic acid) *or* RNA (ribonucleic acid); *never* both. This core is referred to as the **viral genome** and this contains the genetic material which the virus will use to survive and to reproduce itself.

   Viruses are classified as being *either* DNA viruses *or* RNA viruses, depending on the composition of their genome.

Capsid   The genome is enclosed within and intimately attracted to a

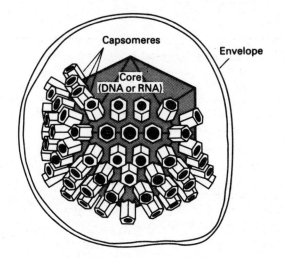

Fig. 2.1 The structure of a virus (with acknowledgement to *Medical Microbiology*, Volume 1, published by Churchill Livingstone)

protein outer shell, known as the **capsid**. The capsid is built from numerous small units **(capsomeres)**.

The capsid serves to protect the delicate nucleic acid of the virus.

Envelope Some viruses are enclosed in a **lipoprotein envelope** (or 'coat'), made up of fat and protein derived from material (nuclear and cytoplasmic membranes) from the cells they infect, which clings to them when they escape, by the process of **budding**.

Virion The genome in the core surrounded by the capsid composes the complete infective viral particle and is known as a **virion**. The virion is the *extra-cellular form of the virus* and can be found prior to the virus entering and taking over another cell. The virion serves as a transportation mechanism, carrying the viral genome to other cells targeted for take-over (i.e. infection).

Viruses are not classified as true cells as they do not contain a limiting plasma membrane, cytoplasm, ribosomes, mitochondria, enzymes to generate high energy bonds, or muramic acid in their outer coverings. However, because they contain nucleic acid, the fundamental property of life, they are able to reproduce, but *only inside another cell*, thus being intracellular parasites.

Shape

The capsid and genome of the virus are closely integrated to form a **nucleocapsid** of an *exactly defined symmetry* (i.e. **shape**).

The capsids of different viruses have different shapes (symmetry). Some are **icosahedral** (cubical) in shape, some are **helical**, and still others are so **complex** that their symmetry has not yet been described. Viruses can be further classified according to their shape, i.e. they are either icosahedral, helical or complex.

Reproduction

Viruses have sometimes been described as 'intracellular parasites' in that they themselves do not possess the intracellular elements necessary to reproduce.

When a virion enters a cell (the **host cell**) it loses its protein capsid (and lipoprotein envelope, if it has one). Viruses use the synthetic machinery in their genome to hijack the nucleus of the cell they have invaded. The viral nucleic acid takes over the genetic material of the host cell, along with the cell's raw materials, energy-producing and metabolic systems. It then reprogrammes the nucleus of the host cell and commands it to produce more viruses: the infected host cell becomes a 'virus factory'. Several hundred new viruses can be produced in each infected host cell which then go on to infect other cells.

Size

Virons are extremely small, varying in diameter from 18 to 300 nanometres (a nanometre (nm) is one-thousandth of a micrometre or one-millionth of a millimetre). There are hundreds of viruses which can infect man. They are usually classified according to their shape, size and the composition of their nucleic acid, i.e. they are either DNA viruses or RNA viruses.

Viral antigenic characters and host cell receptors

Viruses have **antigenic characters** which usually reside in their surface structure. Various types of host cells (i.e. those cells which the virion targets for invasion and take-over) carry **surface receptors** for these antigens to which the virus can bind. The antigenic characters can be thought of as **'keys'** and the host cell receptors as **'locks'**. Each virus which successfully invades man has a key for a certain lock, but not all locks. When a virion enters the human body, it searches for those host cells which have a lock its key will unlock. By using its key, the virus can open the lock and enter ('invade') the cell.

Summary

Viruses are extremely small life forms, being composed of a piece of nucleic acid (either DNA or RNA but not both), the viral genome, surrounded by a protein outer shell (the capsid) and sometimes, in addition, the capsid being surrounded by an envelope made up of fat and protein (lipoprotein). Viruses are of varying but exactly defined shapes and in order to reproduce, must invade and take over the nucleus of another living cell. When viruses invade man, they search for host cells which contain specific surface receptors to which their antigenic characters can bind and then invade the cell. Different viruses have different antigenic characters and as such, are attracted to different host cells. This attraction for specific host cells is known as **tropism**.

Human immunodeficiency viruses

Retroviruses are RNA viruses which have a lipid-containing membrane surrounding the capsid. Retroviruses also have a special viral enzyme, known as **reverse transcriptase**, which allows the virus to make a DNA copy of its RNA genetic material, facilitating its integration into the genetic material of the host cell. Once inserted into the genetic material of the host cell, it directs this cell to produce more RNA retroviruses. Reverse transcriptase refers to the process of making DNA from RNA, the presence of this enzyme being a unique feature of all retroviruses. Although retroviruses were known to cause disease in some animals (leukaemia in cats), it was not thought that they were involved in human disease. In 1978 a new retrovirus, associated with the aetiology of an aggressive, human, adult T cell leukaemia and named **'human T cell leukemia virus'** (HTLV), was isolated by Robert Gallo[6]. In 1982, Gallo identified another similar, but distinct retrovirus from a patient with hairy cell leukaemia. This was named **human T cell leukemia virus, type II (HTLV-II)**[7]. Human T cell leukemia viruses (HTLV) were especially (but not exclusively) attracted to T lymphocytes of the helper subgroup, which became their targets. This attraction (tropism) for helper cells, made them likely candidates for investigation into the aetiology of AIDS as it was known that patients with this disease had a decreased number of helper cells. The possibility that a retrovirus of the HTLV group was involved in the aetiology of AIDS was first reported by Robert Gallo in February 1982[8]. This was followed by Luc Montagnier's discovery of the **lymphadenopathy-associated virus (LAV)** in 1983, and Gallo's discovery of the new type of **human T cell leukaemia virus, type III (HTLV-III)**. In 1984, Dr. Jay Levy in San Francisco also identified the AIDS virus, which he named the **AIDS-associated retrovirus (ARV)**. It is now clear that all of these viruses are different isolates of the same virus.

Special characteristics of HIV

HIV is a retrovirus, 100–120 nanometres in diameter. It is icosahedral in shape which in turn contains a helical nucleocapsid. The genome of HIV is composed of a double strand of RNA and contains many genes which give directions (i.e., **encodes**) to either make viral proteins or are involved in regulating viral replication. The important viral genes are: **env** (encodes the glycoproteins in the viral envelope), **gag** (encodes the core proteins in the virus, e.g. p24, p18), **pol** (encodes viral enzymes, e.g. reverse transcriptase). Viral genes which are important in replication are: **tat** and **rev**, which when switched on, increase viral replication, and **nef**, which when activated, suppresses HIV replication. Surrounding the viral genome is a double protein coat which is itself surrounded by a fatty membrane (lipid bilayer) with sugars (glycoproteins) attached to and imbedded in it. This fatty membrane is the viral envelope (See Fig. 2.2).

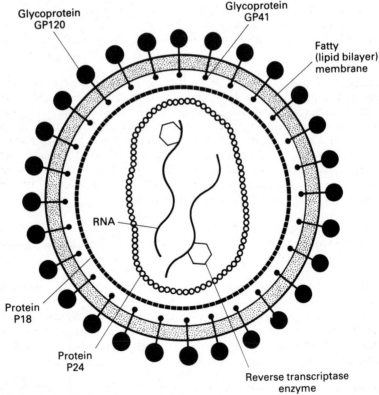

Fig. 2.2   The human immunodeficiency virus (HIV)

The proteins which make up the inner-most coat surrounding the viral genome are termed **p24** (protein weighing 24–25 kilodaltons, sometimes called **p25**). The outer coat of protein is termed **p18** (protein weighing 17–18 kilodaltons and consequently is sometimes referred to as **p17**). These are the core structural proteins. The inner layer of glycoproteins are known as **gp41** and the outer-most layer of glycoproteins are known as **gp120**.

Pathophysiology of HIV infection

The attack

Stage 1:   Targeting for invasion.   The outer glycoproteins, gp120, act as the antigenic 'keys' which are attracted to special host cell receptors ('locks') known as **CD4**. The HIV gp120 allows the virus to bind to the **CD4 host cell receptor**. Host cells which contain the CD4 surface receptors include some lymphocytes (e.g. T4-helper cells), some macrophages and microglial cells in the brain. HIV is commonly referred to as a **lymphotropic virus** because of its attraction to T4 lymphocytes.

Stage 2:   Cell invasion.   The virus, once bound to the host cell CD4 receptors, gains entry into the cell in one of two ways. Cells constantly take in new materials by a process of **endocytosis**, i.e. the cell membrane folds inwards to form a tiny vesicle which carries the material, or in this case, the virus, inside the cell. Eventually the vesicle carrying the virus releases it into the cytoplasm of the host cell. Alternatively, once the gp120 of the virus is locked on to the CD4 receptor, the virus might simply **fuse** its surrounding membrane with the membrane of the cell and quickly enter the cytoplasm of the host cell.

State 3:   Shedding the viral coats.   Either way, once inside the host cell, the viral structure disintegrates, releasing the RNA and the reverse transcriptase enzymes.

Stage 4:   Making the master copy.   Using the reverse transcriptase enzymes, the viral genome *copies itself from RNA to DNA genetic material*. The presence of the enzyme reverse transcriptase and the ability of the viral genome to copy itself from RNA to DNA is a fundamental characteristic of all retroviruses and distinguishes them from other viruses.

Stage 5:   Entering the nucleus.   The viral DNA then enters the nucleus of the host cell and becomes intimately incorporated into the host cell's own DNA. The virus has thus become a *permanent* part of an infected person's own cell.

Stage 6:   The calm before the storm. A period of calm (latency) now ensues and the virus, as it was, ceases to exist. However, the original infective virus has become a latent **provirus** which is sitting in the nucleus of the infected cell awaiting an external signal to start reproducing.

Stage 7:   Viral replication. Chemical signals arrive at the host cell which stimulate it. These signals may be the result of a new infection and would normally result in the cell reproducing itself. However, the nucleus is now reprogrammed by the provirus and instead, reacts to these stimulating signals by manufacturing more virus.

Stage 8:   Cell exit. As more and more viruses are manufactured within the infected cell, they eventually explode outwards, through the cytoplasmic membrane of the host cell by a process known as **budding**. As they leave the infected cell, they surround themselves with protein, lipid and glycoprotein coats which they hijack from the cytoplasmic membranes of the host cell. Once released into the blood stream, they start searching for new target cells which have the special **CD4 lock** and the cycle starts all over again.

Stage 9:   Cell death. The process of new viruses budding out of the original infected host cell causes holes to be punched into the cell membrane of the host cell. Through these holes, essential cellular ingredients escape through the sieve-like membrane until the cell can no longer survive.

Other cells in the immune system may also destroy host cells that were damaged by the budding out of new viruses (an **autoimmune response**).

Summary

HIV has a special affinity for helper cells and infects some but certainly not all of them. Those infected are turned into virus-producing cells and eventually destroyed. Viral replication increases when the infected T-helper cell is activated. Helper cells can be activated by infections (e.g. sexually transmitted diseases) or by the presence of substances containing non-infective antigens such as the antigenic components of concentrated Factor VIII. Newly produced viruses are liberated by 'budding' out from the host cell and infect more helper cells, eventually leading to their destruction. The presence of HIV in some helper cells may also provoke an autoimmune response against non-infected helper cells, causing further destruction of these important cells[9].

Once helper cells are depleted, B lymphocytes are inefficient as they require the 'help' of helper cells to produce specific antibody. Cytotoxic T cell and lymphokine-producing T cell activity is also impaired, resulting in a decreased ability of the immune system to destroy neoplastic and virus infected cells. Some macrophages, which also have special receptors, similar to those found on helper cells (T4 antigens) may be directly infected by HIV.

A sinister feature of HIV infection is the evidence that some cells in the brain (glial cells) are also directly infected[10], causing encephalopathy in patients with AIDS. More ominously, the fact that HIV can infect and slowly replicate within brain cells indicates that this retrovirus belongs to a subfamily known as **lentiviruses**. An infamous member of this subfamily is the **visna virus** which causes a slowly progressive central nervous system deterioration in sheep. In addition to causing a mal-function of the immune system, HIV also causes a parallel central and peripheral nervous system disease, resulting in a variety of neurological dysfunctions, the most common being a progressive dementia associated with a subacute encephalopathy. Should significant numbers of individuals who are currently asymptomatically infected with HIV succumb to neurological disease, the seriousness of this epidemic would take on chilling new features.[11,12]

The origins of the virus

It may be that the exact origins of AIDS will never be completely elicited. There are, however, certain facts that have led to a more or less general agreement as to the source of this epidemic. It is plausible to conclude that HIV is a pathogen new to the human race, probably resulting from a non-pathogenic primate retrovirus, which made a 'species jump' from old world primates (monkeys) to humans. There is widespread evidence that green monkeys in Africa have been infected with a virus similar to HIV for many years[13], although it does not cause disease in these animals. This virus is referred to as **Simian Immunodeficiency Virus (SIV)**. This retrovirus is most likely the progenitor agent from which HIV either mutated or recombined into the human population. Cases of AIDS in Africa became known at about the same time (1981) as American and European cases, although it is likely that human HIV infection existed in Africa long before the disease was recognised. AIDS is now epidemic in some central and east African countries (Zambia, Zaïre, Rwanda, Uganda, and parts of Tanzania). The current pandemic may have started in Africa and have

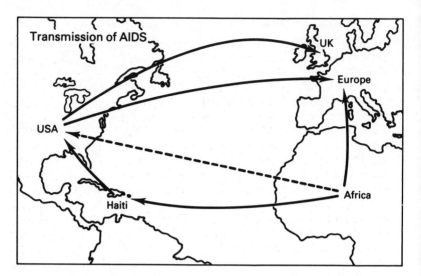

Fig. 2.3   The spread of HIV

spread simultaneously to the USA, Haiti and Europe. Certainly many Haitians lived in Zaire from the early 1960s to the middle 1970s, and then moved to the United States, Europe, or returned to Haiti. It is likely that the spread of AIDS into the UK occurred via British tourists returning from American holidays. However the spread of AIDS into the rest of Europe was more likely a direct result of African links (Fig. 2.3).

Other retroviruses, similar to both SIV and HIV have been identified. Because of this, HIV is now usually referred to as HIV-1. Clavel *et al.* isolated a second type of HIV, referred to as **HIV-2** which originated from the west coast of Africa. HIV-2 is infrequently identified in Europe and the United States, however like HIV-1, does cause AIDS and AIDS-related conditions. It is probable that HIV-2 is the progenitor virus from which HIV-1 emerged and there is probably a continuum of human retroviruses (HTLV-I, HTLV-II, HIV-2, HIV-1) which have developed and show variations in their characteristics. HIV itself shows marked 'antigenic drift', i.e. it is capable of changing its antigenic proteins and producing new 'strains', much like the influenza virus. Intense research is continuing into the origins of the putative progenitor virus of this disease, as new information may lead to a more effective treatment strategy and could lead to the development of an effective vaccine.

Incubation period

As stated previously, HIV is a retrovirus belonging to a sub-group of retroviruses known as lentiviruses. All lentivirus ('slow virus') infections, including HIV infection, are associated with a long incubation period. The incubation period refers to the time between exposure (i.e., day 1 – becoming infected with HIV) to the day when an individual becomes clinically unwell as a result of infection and meets the CDC Case Definition for AIDS. The average incubation period for HIV-1 may be in excess of eleven years, and for HIV-2, it may be seventeen years or longer. However, it is important to remember that some individuals may have a much shorter incubation period (i.e., 'rapid tempo' disease) while others may have a much longer incubation period. Although it is now known that most individuals with HIV infection will eventually become unwell as a result of that infection, there will be cases of individuals who never display any clinical signs or symptoms of HIV infection. The variation among individuals in the incubation period and the eventual consequences of HIV infection may be related to infection with more virulent (or less virulent) strains of HIV or many different co-factors that govern eventual disease expression. Co-factors may include latent infection with other viruses (e.g. Herpes viruses) or a genetic predisposition to ultimate disease expression.

References

1. Auerbach, D.M., Bennett, J.V., Brachman, P.J. and the CDC Task Force. (1982). Epidemiologic aspects of the current outbreak of Kaposi's sarcoma and opportunistic infections. *New England Journal of Medicine* (January 26), 306(4):248–52
2. Gazzard, B.G., Farthing, C., *et al.* (1984). Clinical findings and serological evidence of HTLV-III infections in homosexual contacts of patients with AIDS and Persistent Generalised Lymphadenopathy. *Lancet* (September 1), ii(8401):480–83
3. Barre-Sinoussi, F., Chermann, J.C., *et al.* (1983). Isolation of a T-lymphotropic retrovirus from a patient at risk from acquired immune deficiency syndrome (AIDS). *Science* (May 20), 220(4599):868–71
4. Gallo, R.C., Salahuddin, S.Z., *et al.* (1984). Frequent detection and isolation of cytopathic retroviruses (HTLV-III) from patients with AIDS and at risk from AIDS. *Science* (May 4), 224(4648):500-3
5. Levy, J.A., Hoffman, A.D., *et al.* (1984). Isolation of lymphocytopathic retroviruses from San Francisco patients with AIDS. *Science*, 225:840
6. Poiesz, B.J., Ruscetti, F.W., *et al.* (1980). Detection and isolation of type-C retrovirus particles from fresh and cultured lymphocytes of a patient with cutaneous T-cell lymphoma. *Proceedings of the National Academy of Science* (USA), 77:7415–19

7.   Kalyanaraman, V.S., Sarngaddharan, M.G., *et al.* (1982). A new subtype of human T-cell leukemia virus (HTLV-II) associated with a T-cell variant of hairy cell leukemia. *Science*, 218:571–73

8.   Gallo, R.C., Essex, M. and Gross, L. (1982). *Human T-cell leukemia/lymphoma virus*. Cold Spring Harbor Press, New York, 1984

9.   Bach, J.F. (1988) Mechanisms and pathogenic significance of auto-immunity in AIDS, in *Autoimmune Aspects of HIV Infection*, ed. by Andrieu, J.M., Bach, J.F., Even, P., pp 1–5, Royal Society of Medicine Services, Ltd., London

10. Levy, J.A., Hollander, H., *et al.* (1985). Isolation of AIDS-associated retroviruses from cerebrospinal fluid and brain of patients with neuro-logical symptoms. *Lancet*. (September 14), ii(8455):568–8

11. Rosenblum, M.L., Levy, R.M. and Bredesen, D.E. (1988). *AIDS and the Nervous System*, Raven Press, New York

12. Price, R.W. and Brew, B. (1990). Management of the Neurological Complications of HIV-1 Infection and AIDS, in *The Medical Management of AIDS*, 2nd ed., pp 161–181, ed. by Sande, M.A. and Volberding, P.A., W.B. Saunders Co., London

13. Biggar, R.J. (1986). The AIDS Problem in Africa, *Lancet* (January 11), i(8472):79–83

Further Reading

Levy, J.A. (1990) Features of HIV and the Host Response that Influence Progression to Disease, in, *The Medical Management of AIDS*, 2nd ed., pp 161–181, ed. by Sande, M.A. and Volberding, P.A., W.B. Saunders Co., London

Cann, A.J. and Karn, J. (1989). Molecular biology of HIV: new insights into the virus life-cycle, *AIDS*, 3(Suppl1):S19–S34

3

The Immunological Background to the Acquired Immune Deficiency Syndrome

An understanding of normal immune mechanisms is necessary in order to appreciate fully the immune dysfunctions seen in AIDS. Immunity, an increased resistance to infectious disease, has evolved in man over the centuries and affords essential protection, without which survival would be impossible. There are many non-specific mechanisms available to everyone, which we employ to protect ourselves against infection – non-specific in that they are used to attack all potential pathogens (microbes which cause disease). This type of immunity, referred to as **innate** immunity, is geared towards either the prevention of pathogenic invasion or containment and eventual resolution should invasion occur.

Prevention of invasion

Intact skin. A healthy, intact skin provides a good barrier against invasion by pathogens. It is unusual, however, for skin to be perfectly intact as all of us have small or microscopic abrasions. At any rate, sweat glands, hair follicles, etc., provide an entry for many potential pathogens.

Mucous membranes and ciliated cells. External openings of the body are guarded by mucous membranes. For example, the mouth, nose, urethra, vagina and rectum are all lined with mucous membranes. These membranes secrete sticky mucus so that when pathogens enter the body by one of these routes, many of them are impinged on these sticky, mucous surfaces. Many of these membranes are associated with cells, which have hair-like processes, known as **cilia** (e.g. the upper respiratory system) which are then able to waft pathogens away from deeper structures, eventually assisting in expelling them from the body.

pH changes. Some areas of the body have a pH which is often hostile to many pathogens. For example, the pH of the vagina is acid and pathogens which require an alkaline medium to reproduce would not be successful in establishing infection in this environment. The pH changes in the gastro-intestinal tract, where ingested food is first mixed with saliva in an alkaline medium in the mouth, is then swallowed into the acid environment of the stomach, and eventually passed into the alkaline environment of the duodenum, can be either bacteriostatic (preventing bacterial growth) or bacteriocidal (killing bacteria) to many pathogens.

Chemical secretions. Many secretions in the body can be either bacteriocidal or -static. For example, nasal secretions, saliva, sweat and tears all contain substances known as **lysozymes**, which are bacteriocidal to many Gram-positive bacteria. In the presence of **complement**, lysozymes can destroy many Gram-negative bacteria. Another substance in serum is **properdin** which is also able to destroy many Gram-negative bacteria and (with complement) many viruses.

Containment of invading pathogens

Effective as these non-specific mechanisms are, pathogenic invasion does occur from time to time. The body still has some fairly sophisticated, non-specific mechanisms available to deal with these pathogens, which, if successful, contain them, limit the damage and eventually destroy them. These include:

Inflammation – this is a protective mechanism, which results in an increase in local blood supply to the area under attack. This hyperaemia is the cause of the classic signs of inflammation (heat, redness, swelling and pain). With this increased blood supply come cells which are able to engage in *phagocytosis*.

Phagocytosis – the normal white blood cell count is made up of different white cells which have different functions. In every cubic millimetre of blood, there are between 8000 and 10 000 white blood cells – this is referred to as a normal **white cell count**. Making up this total white cell count are:
(i)   **Polymorphonuclear white blood cells (granulocytes).**
      These account for 70 per cent of the white cells
      There are 3 different types of polymorphonuclear cells: **basophils, eosinophils and neutrophils**
      Neutrophils account for most of the polymorphs and are actively phagocytic (basophils and eosinophils are not phagocytic cells – they have different functions)
(ii) **Monocytes.** These make up 5 per cent of the white cell count and these cells are also phagocytic
(iii) **Lymphocytes.** These make up the remaining 25 per cent of the white cell count – these cells are not phagocytic and will be

discussed later. There are two different types of lymphocytes: **T cells** and **B cells**

Phagocytosis is the process by which bacteria are engulfed by neutrophils and monocytes and eventually destroyed. Other cells in the body capable of phagocytosis are known as **macrophages**.

Other determinants of innate immunity which influence the ability of the individual to withstand infectious disease include:

Nutrition – a well nourished individual is better able to deal with an infectious process than people who are not well nourished.

Age – the very young and the very old are less able to ward off infectious diseases.

Race – some races are either more prone to or more immune from certain diseases than others.

Species – man is immune to many of the diseases which affect animals and vice versa.

All of these factors, associated with innate immunity, offer good protection against infectious diseases. However, by themselves, they are not adequate for survival in the hostile environment in which man finds himself. We need much more specific protection and this is afforded by the specific immune response of acquired immunity.

Acquired immunity – the specific immune response

During the first few months of life, the infant begins to acquire protection against specific pathogens. This type of immunity, known as **acquired immunity**, allows the child to mount a **specific immune response** towards each pathogen the child encounters as it progresses through those first vulnerable months and years. For the first three months of its life, the child is protected by the natural, passive immunity conferred by the mother. During these first few months, antibodies from the mother pass to the child while it is still in the uterus. However, these antibodies are short-lived and by the end of three months, the child must begin to acquire its own immunity.

Acquired immunity involves two different but interrelated processes. The first process is known as humoral immunity.

Humoral immunity

The active agents of acquired immunity are the lymphocytes. We have already mentioned that there are two different types of lymphocytes – the **B lymphocytes** and the **T lymphocytes**. Both originate from stem cells, which are manufactured in the bone marrow. Some of these stem cells, destined to become B lymphocytes (B cells) are known as B cell precursors. The remaining stem cells, destined to become T lymphocytes are, of course, T cell precursors. The B cell precursors migrate back to the bone marrow, where they are 'processed' into B lymphocytes. They are known as B lymphocytes as they were first identified in the hindgut of a bird, an area known as the 'Bursa of Fabricius'. Although humans do not have this special tissue, it is thought that they have similar areas (Bursa equivalent areas), such as the foetal liver and the bone marrow, which 'process' B cell precursors in such a way that when they develop into fully mature B lymphocytes, they respond in a specific manner to pathogens. The manner in which they respond is known as **humoral immunity**. B lymphocytes account for about 30 per cent of all lymphocytes (the remaining 70 per cent being T lymphocytes). Figure 3.1 illustrates the development of a mature B lymphocyte.

Humoral immunity is acquired as follows: a foreign cell, be it a bacterium, a virus, a tissue cell, etc., is recognized by the body as 'not self' and referred to as an **antigen**. For the moment, we are going to think of antigens as bacteria or viruses, but they can be anything (usually a protein) which the body detects as 'different'. These antigens are 'pre-processed' by phagocytic cells and eventually present to the B lymphocytes in lymphatic tissue (e.g. spleen, liver, bone marrow and lymph nodes) where the presence of this antigen stimulates the B cell to proliferate and change into **plasma cells** and **memory cells**. Plasma cells have a specific function which is to secrete a protein substance known as **antibody**. The rate of antibody secretion is impressive, in the order of 2000 antibody molecules per second for each plasma cell. This goes on for several days until the plasma cell dies (4–5 days).

The antibody then combines with antigen. This combination of antibody plus antigen equals an **immune complex**. Antibodies protect the individual in several ways: firstly, the antibody attacks the antigen's cell wall, weakening and eventually destroying it; this is known as lysis.

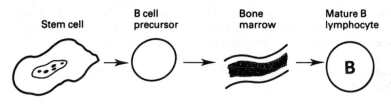

| Stem cell | B cell precursor | Bone marrow | Mature B lymphocyte |

Fig. 3.1   The maturation of a B lymphocyte

More importantly, when the antibody 'coats' or attaches itself to an antigen, the formation of immune complexes sets off a cascade of chemical events in which certain enzymes in the blood (complement enzymes) become activated in a sequential manner, resulting in active **complement**. Complement has two important functions: it initiates a local inflammatory reaction at the invasion site, which increases the local blood supply, and secondly, by-products of inflammation chemically attract neutrophils, monocytes and other phagocytic cells known as **macrophages** (discussed later) to the area under attack. This chemical attraction of phagocytic cells to the invasion site is known as **chemotaxis**. Some antigens are destroyed by direct cell wall damage when coated by complement.

We can see that it is critically important for plasma cells to secrete antibody. There are two important points to remember: the antibody produced is specific to that particular antigen, for example if the antigen was the chickenpox virus, then the antibody produced would bind only to the chickenpox virus – it would not bind to the measles virus. Secondly, antibody is formed in a sequential manner, something like: antibody 1, antibody 2, antibody 3, etc. Hence, soon after invasion, antibody 1 is formed, then in a week or so, antibody 2 is formed, and so on. If we took a sample of blood at week two of the infection, we might find the first antibody still there, but disappearing, and the second antibody just appearing. Perhaps antibody 1 would disappear within a month but antibody 2 would stay in the serum for years, or for life. This would be important, as the presence of antibody 1 would be a diagnostic marker of acute infection while antibody 2 would be a marker of previous exposure. However, all the antibodies would be antibodies to that specific antigen (e.g. the chickenpox virus) – they would simply be different classes of the antibody.

All the different classes of antibodies are collectively known as **immunoglobulins**. They are not of course called antibody 1, antibody 2, etc., but rather IgM, IgG, IgA, IgD and IgE (the 'Ig' stands for immunoglobulin – hence, the classes of immunoglobulin are M, G, A, D, and E). A few points about the different classes of immunoglobulins:

IgM – this important class of antibody usually appears early in the course of an infectious disease and disappears as the patient recovers. **Hence it is a marker of acute infection**. It accounts for about six per cent of the total amount of immunoglobulin formed and works by neutralizing pathogens (especially viruses) by lysis or by enhancing phagocytosis.

IgG (gamma-globulin) – this class of antibody accounts for 70–90 per cent of all the immunoglobulin formed, being especially useful at activating complement and promoting phagocytosis. It remains in the body for long periods of time (years, or a lifetime) hence **its presence is not an indication of acute infection, but rather of previous exposure.**

IgA – accounts for up to 13 per cent of the total amount of immunoglobulin formed, but accounts for over 90 per cent of the immunoglobulin found on mucosal surfaces (e.g. nose, mouth) and protects the body by neutralizing antigens that enter by these routes.

IgD – accounts for about 18 per cent of the total amount of immunoglobulin formed – not much is known for certain about its specific function.

IgE – only accounts for about 0.002 per cent of immunoglobulin formed and this can bind to 'mast cells' causing these cells to release vasoactive substances, such as histamine and serotonin, which are responsible for the common signs and symptoms of acute allergic reactions.

Memory cells – when provoked by the presence of an antigen, both T cells and B cells produce **memory cells**, clones of the stimulated parent cell. Should the individual encounter the same antigen any time in the future, the cascade of events which constitute a specific immune response will be accelerated. This is because memory cells 'remember' the specific antigen and respond quickly.

Mast cells – these are special cells, which are capable of releasing substances such as heparin, histamine, serotonin and SRS (slow-reacting-substance) of anaphylaxis when stimulated to do so by IgE immunoglobulin bound to their surface. One type of polymorphonuclear white blood cell, a basophil, is a type of circulating mast cell – others are 'fixed' in most tissues of the body, for example lung tissue.

Macrophages – these cells ('big eaters') are efficient phagocytic cells and are found permanently attached to loose connective tissue and various organs of the body (i.e. **fixed macrophages**) such as the Kupffer cells of the liver, splenocytes of the spleen, dust cells of the lung, microglia in the spinal cord and brain and histiocytes in loose, connective tissue. Other macrophages wander around the body (i.e. **free macrophages**) and are found in areas of inflammation, having been attracted there by the process of chemotaxis. Macrophages search for foreign invaders and when they locate these antigens, signal a warning to the T lymphocytes, which initiates cell-mediated immunity. Macrophages also attempt to destroy the invading antigen by engulfing them (i.e. phagocytosis). Many macrophages, like T4-helper cells, carry the CD4 receptor on their surface and hence are a target for HIV.

Summary   Humoral immunity is the process whereby B lymphocytes, provoked by the presence of an antigen, proliferate and undergo change, some changing into memory cells, but most changing into plasma cells. Plasma cells have just one function – to secrete specific antibody which can combine with the antigen, forming immune complexes, activating the complement system and by different methods, eventually destroying the invading pathogen.

Cell-mediated immunity

The other process involved in acquired immunity is that of **cell-mediated immunity**. This involves the T lymphocytes which are derived from the same stem cells as B lymphocytes, but which migrate to the **thymus gland** for processing, rather than to bone marrow and other bursa equivalent areas. In the thymus gland, these T cell precursors are 'processed' to react differently when they encounter antigens. Mature T lymphocytes account for about 70 per cent of the total number of lymphocytes. When they encounter an antigen, they differentiate into several different subsets (Fig. 3.3):

Lymphokine producing cells (T-D cells) – these cells release various **lymphokines**, substances which mediate other inflammatory cells and phagocytic cells. Several lymphokines are released by T-D cells, including **interferon** and **interleukin 2**. Interferon has a direct anti-virus effect and also activates a cell known as a **natural killer cell** (NK cell). These cells, once activated, are involved in preventing the development of tumours in the body. If they were defective, there would be an increased incidence of cancer in an individual. Other lymphokines act on other cells, enhancing inflammation and chemotaxis.

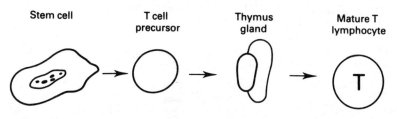

| Stem cell | T cell precursor | Thymus gland | Mature T lymphocyte |

Fig. 3.2   The maturation of a T lymphocyte

Cytotoxic cells (T-C cells) – these important cells are necessary to destroy cells harbouring viruses. They require T-helper cells to activate and any deficiency in cytotoxic cell activity would render the individual at increased risk of viral infections.

Regulator cells – these cells regulate the activity of all the other subsets of both B cells, and T cells. There are two different regulator cells: **helper cells** which 'help' plasma cells effectively secrete specific antibody, 'help' cytotoxic cells activate, and 'help' lymphokine-producing

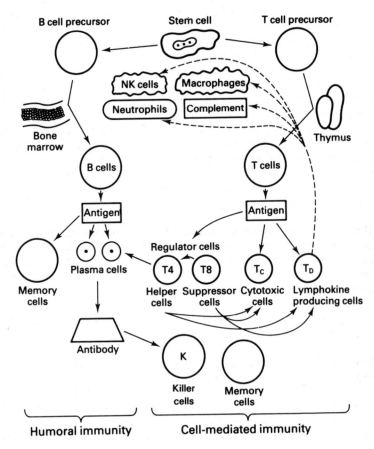

Acquired immunity

Fig. 3.3   Acquired immunity

cells activate and release their various chemical mediators. **Suppressor cells** will eventually 'suppress' helper cells, cytotoxic and lymphokine-producing cells when the emergency is over. Helper cells are also known as **T4 lymphocytes** or **CD4+ lymphocytes** and suppressor cells are known as **T8 lymphocytes or CD8+ lymphocytes**.

Figure 3.3 illustrates the interrelationship between humoral and cell-mediated immunity, and the crucial role played by the helper (T4) cells.

Immune dysfunctions

Survival is impossible without a well-functioning immune system. However, immune dysfunction is clinically well recognised. Some children are born with a **primary immune dysfunction**, such as Severe Combined Immunodeficiency (SCID) or DiGeorge Syndrome. In these conditions, fatal flaws in the immune system render the child unable to mount a specific immune response to invading pathogens. The child will die of infectious diseases, which take the opportunity of establishing themselves in a host who is unable to defend himself effectively – hence these infections are referred to as **opportunistic infections**.

Most individuals, however, are born with an effective and fully functional immune system. As life progresses, events and incidents can occur which may depress the immune system, either temporarily or permanently. These are the immunodeficiencies, which are secondary to another cause or condition, i.e. **secondary immunodeficiency**. Secondary immunodeficiencies can be caused by:

Drugs. Administration of corticosteroids, immunosuppressants, and most anti-cancer drugs will depress the immune system. During this period, the patient is at increased risk of opportunistic infections, a fact well known to nurses as evidenced by their careful monitoring of patients while on this type of treatment.

Malignant conditions. Hodgkin's disease, leukaemia and other malignancies can cause a severe immunodeficiency.

Protein depletion conditions. Antibodies are made up of protein molecules. Any condition in which there is an inadequate supply of protein in the body leads to an immunodeficient state. This can be seen in conditions such as the nephrotic syndrome in which there is a renal loss of protein (especially IgG), and in starvation, where inadequate protein renders the individual (often a child) prone to common infections, such as measles, which may then be rapidly fatal.

Radiation.   Radiation can depress the bone marrow, affecting its ability to produce the stem cells which eventually become fully mature lymphocytes.

Other conditions.   Ageing, debilitation, various infectious diseases, diseases such as sarcoidosis, leprosy, and miliary TB can all cause immunodeficiency, resulting in the individual becoming vulnerable to opportunistic disease.

Immunodeficiency seen in AIDS

AIDS is chiefly, but not exclusively a disorder of cell-mediated immunity. The most striking immunological features seen in AIDS are:

Leucopenia

A reduction in the normal number of white blood cells is accounted for by a severe peripheral **lymphocytopenia**, i.e. a reduction in the numbers of lymphocytes. This reduction in lymphocytes is due to a diminution of helper (T4) cells; suppressor (T8) cells are either unaffected or may increase in number. Regardless, the reduction in helper (T4) cells alters the normal ratio of helper (T4) cells to suppressor (T8) cells (normally 2:1). The normal number of peripheral T4 (CD4+) helper cells is approximately 800–1000 mm^3. In advancing HIV infection, this number can decrease to well under 100 mm^3. A T4 (CD4+) helper cell count of under 500 mm^3 may be an indication for anti-retroviral treatment and a T4 (CD4+) helper cell count of under 200 mm^3 is generally an indication for specific prophylaxis against common infections seen in AIDS. Not only are helper (T4) cells reduced in number, but they are also functionally defective.

Impaired lymphokine production

There is a defective production of some lymphokines (e.g. interleukin 2 and gamma-interferon).

Defective natural killer cell activity

Although there are normal numbers of circulating NK cells, they are defective. This is related to the decreased production of interferons by lymphokine-producing cells and is probably the chief reason why patients with AIDS are particularly susceptible to Kaposi's sarcoma.

Impaired cytotoxic cell activity

In AIDS, defective cell-mediated cytotoxicity against target cells harbouring viruses is seen. Consequently, patients with AIDS are at increased risk of viral infections.

Defective monocyte function

There is both defective chemotaxis and an impaired ability of monocytes to destroy many pathogens (e.g. *Giardia lamblia, Toxoplasma gondii*).

Polyclonal activation of B lymphocytes

Although principally a disease of cell-mediated immunity, B cells are also abnormal, secreting large amounts of non-specific IgG and IgA. As a result, patients with AIDS have elevated levels of gamma-globulin. As the B cells are functionally defective, the antibody produced is undifferentiated, i.e. faulty and non-specific. Patients with AIDS are not able to develop specific humoral immunity to any new antigens.

Summary

It can be appreciated that perhaps the most devastating immunological defect in patients with AIDS is the absolute reduction in helper (T4) cells. Without the 'help' of these cells, the entire, intricate pattern of the immune system is defective. It is thus easier to understand why patients with AIDS present with opportunistic infections and neoplastic conditions. It is this new understanding of these defects of acquired immunity which is pointing the way for many researchers as they quickly move forward in investigating the treatment of this catastrophic condition.

Further reading

1. Pinching, A.J., Weiss, R.A., Miller, D., editors (1988). *AIDS and HIV infection: The Wider Perspective*, British Medical Bulletin, **44**(1), Churchill Livingstone, London.
2. Sande, M.A. and Volberding, P.A. (1990). *The Medical Management of AIDS*, 2nd ed., W.B. Saunders Co., London.

4

The Means of Transmission

The AIDS epidemic is a composite of many individual, though
overlapping, smaller epidemics, each with its own dynamics and
time course.
Morbidity and Mortality Weekly Report 36(49)
18 December, 1987

HIV is a blood-borne virus and has been isolated from blood[1],
semen[2], saliva[3], tears[4], breast milk[5] and cerebrospinal fluid[6]. It is
principally a sexually transmitted disease. However, transmission can
occur via a variety of methods involving contact with blood, blood products, and other body fluids, as listed in Table 4.1.

Table 4.1   HIV: means of transmission

1. Sexually, via contact with infected blood, semen, and cervical and
   vaginal fluids
2. Following transfusion of blood or blood products from donor blood
   infected with HIV
3. Injecting substance misuse – contamination with infected blood
   through sharing needles and syringes
4. Following organ transplants or artificial insemination by donor semen
5. Transplacental and perinatal transmission

Sexual transmission.   The chief route of transmission is via sexual
activity. Homosexual (and heterosexual) anal intercourse is an efficient
means of transmission, due to the presence of both potentially infected
semen and small amounts of blood, which are common in penetrative
rectal intercourse. In Europe and the United States, homosexual or
bisexual men constitute the largest group of individuals who have contracted HIV infection. This is due to the propensity for anal sex and
the multiplicity of sexual partners often associated with this group.
Heterosexual vaginal intercourse is also an efficient means of virus
transmission, due to both potentially infected semen and vaginal and

cervical secretions containing infected lymphocytes. In Africa, AIDS is principally a heterosexually spread disease.

Blood and blood products. HIV has been transmitted following transfusion of whole blood, blood components and the administration of concentrated Factor VIII, manufactured from pooled plasma and used in the treatment of haemophilia. The routine screening of donor blood for the presence of anti-HIV and the self-exclusion of donors who, on the known means of transmission, may have been exposed to HIV, will substantially decrease (but not totally eliminate) infection from this source.

Injecting substance misuse. Individuals who misuse injectable drugs account for the second largest group of individuals who have contracted HIV infection, both in the United States and in Europe. In the European Community (EC), by 1989, the incidence of new AIDS cases among injecting substance misusers had become equal to that occuring among homo/bisexual men and is expected to increase significantly during 1991–92[7]. HIV infection is transmitted by sharing blood-contaminated needles and syringes.

Organ transplants and artificial insemination by donor semen. Donor organs (kidneys, corneas, hearts) are a potential risk and individuals whose previous behaviour has put them at risk of acquiring HIV infection are advised not to donate organs or to carry donor cards. A further risk with donor organ transplantation is that recipients receive immunosuppressive therapy to prevent rejection and frequently receive blood transfusions during surgery. The routine screening of donors for anti-HIV will diminish this risk substantially. Cases have been reported of recipients of artificial insemination of donor semen acquiring HIV infection[8]. This risk will decrease with screening of donors, the voluntary self-exclusion of donors who, on the known means of transmission, may have been exposed to HIV, and the exclusive use of cryopreserved donor semen, stored for 3–6 months and not used until the donor has been retested for anti-HIV. The use of fresh semen in artificial insemination programmes will remain a possible risk.

Transplacental and perinatal transmission. AIDS in children was first reported in 1982. As of March 1990, 2192 children under the age of 13 years in the United States had been diagnosed as suffering from AIDS. Children have contracted HIV infection as a result of receiving blood transfusions or concentrated Factor VIII for haemophilia, or more commonly, as a result of having a parent infected with HIV. Paediatric cases of HIV infection have occurred in the UK and in other European countries (over 800 cases in Europe by the end of 1989). Infection may be contracted *in utero*, at birth, or in the neonatal period. Most cases result from perinatal transmission of HIV[9]. There has been one documented case of a child, infected by blood transfusions, who transmitted the infection to his mother who frequently became contaminated with blood and body fluids when caring for him[10].

Transmission categories

In both the UK and the USA, most cases of AIDS (80% in the UK and 60% in the USA) have occurred in men with homosexual or bisexual orientation. This transmission group is often referred to as the '**First Wave**' of the epidemic and it is important to remember that because of the long incubation period of AIDS, the current cases of gay men with AIDS only reflects what was happening ten to fifteen years ago. There is now convincing evidence that many homosexual men started changing their sexual behaviour as early as mid-1987 and the numbers of gay men becoming infected with HIV started to decline at that time[11]. Whether or not this change in behaviour can be sustained is not certain.

The '**Second Wave**' of the epidemic involves individuals who misuse injectable drugs. In both Europe and the USA, this transmission group is accounting for an ever increasing number of both individuals who are infected with HIV and those with symptomatic disease as a result of HIV infection[12]. It is important to remember that individuals who misuse injectable drugs are generally sexually active (both heterosexually and homosexually) and it is usually impossible to ascertain exactly how they became infected. However, it is acknowledged that sharing blood contaminated injecting equipment is a more efficient means of viral transmission than sexual intercourse.

Finally, the '**Third Wave**' of the epidemic involves men and women who have been become infected with HIV as a result of heterosexual exposure[13]. As more women become infected, more perinatally infected infants will be born.

During the 1990s, individuals from the second and third waves of the epidemic will come to dominate the numbers of patients/clients requiring nursing care as a result of symptomatic HIV infection.

Transmission categories are different in the various parts of the world affected by this pandemic. The World Health Organisation has described three epidemiological patterns of spread. **Pattern I** countries are those (e.g. Europe, USA) in which the predominant mode of transmission is among homosexual or bisexual males and injecting substance misusers. **Pattern II** countries are those (e.g. sub-Saharan Africa) in which the predominant means of transmission is from heterosexual exposure. Some countries (e.g. Latin America and the Caribbean) demonstrate a combination of Pattern I and Pattern II transmission models. However, they seem to be evolving towards a Pattern II model. **Pattern III** countries (e.g. China, India) are those who report only a small number of cases, many of which are imported. It is likely that many Pattern III countries will evolve into a Pattern II situation.

Globally, the vast majority of individuals who have become infected with HIV have done so as a result of heterosexual exposure[14].

Sexual transmission of HIV, in both the USA and the UK, is most frequently **male-to-male** and is well documented. **Male-to-female transmission** is also well documented by accounts of HIV infection in women after artificial insemination with donor semen and by haemophiliacs who have passed HIV infection to their wives. Indeed, there is one documented case of a woman contracting AIDS as a result of a single episode of vaginal intercourse[15]. **Female-to-male transmission**, occurs as evidenced by the current situation in Africa, where there are equal numbers of men and women infected, and the documentation of clusters of heterosexual cases[16]. Prostitutes, many of whom are injecting substance misusers, may well become a reservoir of infection and an important 'bridging group' in the future. **Female-to-female** transmission is reported from time to time but must be extremely rare[17].

Male-to-male (via anal intercourse) and male-to-female (via vaginal or anal intercourse) are the two most efficient means of sexually transmitting HIV. Female-to-male and passive male-to-active male (during anal intercourse) transmission is less effecient because the concentration of virus (i.e., the number of 'infectious particles per million' or ppm) is generally higher in semen than in vaginal or cervical secretions. However, an increased number of white cells in cervical or vaginal secretions (as seen in chronic pelvic inflammatory diseases, e.g. sexually transmitted diseases) or the presence of even small amounts of blood will enhance the effectiveness of female-to-male (or passive-male-to-active male during anal intercourse) viral transmission.

Risk factors

Other factors involved in the probability of effecient sexual transmission of HIV include:

Type of sexual activity   Penetrative vaginal and anal intercourse, sexual intercourse during the menstrual cycle and the number of times an individual has unprotected penetrative intercourse with an infected partner all increase the likelihood of viral transmission. Passive (i.e., receptive) vaginal and anal intercourse are significantly associated with a higher risk of HIV acquisition than active (i.e., insertive) intercourse. Oral-genital sex has not been conclusively associated with HIV transmission but active anal-oral sex ('rimming') may be associated with the transmission of an oncogenic agent which may cause Kaposi's sarcoma[18]. Deep, passionate kissing ('French kissing') has also not conclusively been shown to be associated with HIV transmission.

Disease stage of the index case (i.e., the infected partner)   It is probable that an infected individual is most infectious, from a sexual transmission point of view, shortly after becoming infected and then after a long period of time when they become unwell as a result of that infection. Infectiousness in the index case may be associated with a positive HIV culture and/or the presence of p24 antigen.

Viral variants   HIV shows great abilities towards 'antigenic drift' and it is possible that some viral strains are more virulent than others.

Presence of other sexually transmitted diseases (STDs)   Not only do other concurrent STDs recruit additional white cells and macrophages to the sexual field, but they may also alter the protective mucosa of the vagina, rectum or urethra, increasing the probability of HIV transmission. This is especially true of ulcerative STDs, e.g. genital herpes, chancroid and primary syphilis.

Viral load   The amount of virus to which an individual is exposed is significant. Being exposed to a large amount of virus not only increases the risk of ultimately being infected but may also lead to an accelerated progression into fully expressed AIDS[19].

Lack of male circumcision   If the male is uncircumcised, there is a greater probability of viral acquisition than in circumcised men[20].

Bleeding during sex   Any open lesions, however small, which result from trauma during sexual activity, may result in bleeding which would increase the likelihood of both transmission and acquisition of HIV.

Number of sexual partners   A direct relationship exists between the number of different sexual partners and the probability of contracting HIV infection during unprotected, penetrative sexual activity.

   Although homosexual men were particularly vulnerable to this infection during the early years of the epidemic, AIDS and other manifestations of HIV infection are not exclusive to this group of individuals. All sexually active individuals can be infected, if exposed to the virus under the right circumstances. Nurses have both a unique responsibility and opportunity to assist in the health education efforts currently being implemented by the Health Services aimed at primary prevention. The role of the nurse in patient education as related to HIV infection is discussed in Chapter 12.

References

1. Gallo, R.C., Salahuddin, S.Z., Popovic, M., *et al.* (1984). Frequent detection and isolation of cytopathic retroviruses (HTLV-III) from patients with AIDS and at risk for AIDS. *Science*, 224:500–3
2. Zagury, D., Bernard, J., Leibowitch, J., *et al.* (1984). HTLV-III in cells cultured from semen of two patients with AIDS. *Science*, 226:449–51
3. Groopman, J.E., Salahuddin, S.Z., Sarngadharan, M.G., *et al.* (1984). HTLV-III in saliva of people with AIDS-related complex and healthy homosexual men at risk for AIDS. *Science*, 226:447–9
4. Fujikawa, L.S., Palestine, A.G., Nussenblatt, R.B., *et al.* (1985). Isolation of human T-lymphotropic virus type III from the tears of a patient with the Acquired Immune Deficiency Syndrome. *Lancet*, (September 7), ii(8454):529–30
5. Thirty, L., Sprecher-Goldberger, S., Jonckheer, T., *et al.* (1985). Isolation of AIDS virus from cell-free breast milk of three healthy virus carriers. *Lancet* (October 19), ii(8460):891–2
6. Levy, J.A., Hollander, H., Shimabukura, J., *et al.* (1985). Isolation of AIDS-associated retroviruses from cerebrospinal fluid and brain of patients with neurological symptoms. *Lancet* (September 14), ii(8455):586–8
7. Downs, A. (1990), *Europe: WHO Predictions to 1991*, Abstracts, VI International Conference on AIDS, San Francisco, USA
8. Steward, G.J., Cunningham, A.L., Driscoll, G.L., *et al.* (1985). Transmission of Human T-Cell Lymphotropic Virus Type III (HTLV-III) by artificial insemination by donor semen. *Lancet* (September 14) ii(8455):581–4
9. Quinn, T.C. (1990). Global Epidemiology of HIV Infections, in *The Medical Management of AIDS*, ed. Sande, M.A. and Volberding, P.A., pp 13–14, W.B. Saunders Co., London
10. Centers for Disease Control (1986) Apparent transmission of Human T-Lymphotropic Virus Type II/Lymphadenopathy-Associated Virus from a child to a mother providing health care, *MMWR*, 35(5):76–9
11. Centers for Disease Control (1990). Update: acquired immunodeficiency syndrome – United States, 1989, *MMWR*, **39**:81–6
12. WHO (1989). *AIDS Surveillance in Europe*, WHO Collaborating Centre on AIDS, Quarterly report, 31 December
13. Rowen, D. and Carne, C.A. (1990). Heterosexual transmission of human immunodeficiency virus, *International Journal of STD and AIDS* (July) **1**(4):239–244
14. Alexander, N.J., Gabelnick, H.L., Spieler, J.M., eds. (1990). *Heterosexual Transmission of AIDS*, Wiley-Liss, New York, USA

15. Cabane, J., Thibierge, E., Godeau, P. *et al*. (1984). AIDS in an apparently risk-free woman, *Lancet* (July 14), ii(8394):105
16. Alexander, N.J., Gabelnick, H.L., Spieler, J.M., *op. cit.*
17. Edwards, A. & Thin, R.N. (1990). Sexually transmitted diseases in lesbians, *International Journal of STD and AIDS*, (May) 1(3):178–181
18. Jacobson, L., Munoz, A., Dudley, J., *et al*. for the Multicenter AIDS Cohort Study MACS (1990). *Examination of timing of potential Kaposi's sarcoma cofactor relative to HIV-1 infection*, VI Internation Conference on AIDS, 1990, San Francisco, Abstracts TH.C.631
19. Schechter, M.T., Craib, K.J.P., Le, T.N., *et al*. (1990). Susceptibility to AIDS progression appears early in HIV infection, *AIDS* (March), 4(3):185–190
20. Alexander, N.J., Gabelnick, H.L., Spieler, J.M., *op. cit.*

5

The Presenting Illnesses of Acquired Immunodeficiency Syndrome

> A succession of disasters came on him so swiftly and with such
> unexpected violence that it is hard to say when exactly I recognized
> that my friend was in deep trouble.
>
> *Brideshead Revisited.* Evelyn Waugh

The clinical presentation of HIV infection

In August 1987, the Centers for Disease Control (CDC) in Atlanta
published their latest case definition of AIDS[1] and this is reproduced in
Appendix 1.

It may be that everyone infected with HIV will eventually develop
some form of ill health as a result of infection. HIV infection is a
dynamic process incorporating various phases, which are illustrated in
Fig. 5.1.

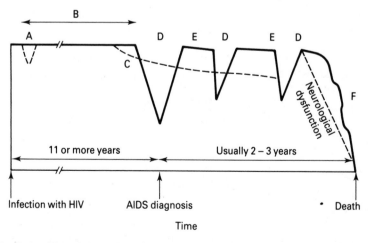

Fig. 5.1 Clinical dynamics of HIV infection

Phase A: Acute seroconversion illness

As previously mentioned in Chapter 2, some (but not all) individuals develop an acute 'glandular fever like illness' two to six weeks after primary or initial infection with HIV. This is characterized by fever, joint pains (arthralgias), tenderness and pain in the muscles (myalgias), diarrhoea and a maculopapular rash. Individuals may also develop a variety of self-limiting neurological manifestations of acute HIV infection, for example atypical aseptic meningitis and acute encephalitis and these are discussed in more detail in Chapter 6. Some individuals develop generalized swollen lymph glands (lymphadenopathy) in response to acute HIV infection, which resolve in several weeks[2]. During this time, the infected individual will start to produce antibodies to HIV (i.e. seroconversion). This acute reaction to HIV infection may go unrecognized in many individuals.

Phase B: Antibody positive phase

Following seroconversion, the infected individual becomes antibody positive and may remain asymptomatic for many years prior to developing clinical illness as a result of infection. This phase of infection can be subdivided into:

Phase B-1: Asymptomatic HIV infection

Many individuals infected with HIV remain clinically asymptomatic (at least in the first 11–12 year period). However, several laboratory abnormalities characteristic of overt disease may be found in these individuals. These laboratory abnormalities are described in Table 5.1.

As infection progresses, leucopenia may become more serious and a reduction in lymphocytes (lymphocytopenia) can develop. A reduction in thrombocytes (thrombocytopenia) may also be seen but is not usually associated with bleeding unless aggravated by a drug reaction, for example trimethoprim-sulfamethoxazole ('Septrin')[3].

The majority of people in this group are unidentified. By the end of 1990, almost 50 000 individuals in England and Wales will be asympto-

Table 5.1　Laboratory abnormalities in acute HIV infection

1.　Depressed T-helper (T4) cell number and function
2.　Raised immunoglobulin levels
3.　Leucopenia (white blood cells $<5.0 \times 10^9/1$). (Differential count, i.e. percentage of different types of white blood cells, is usually normal in the early or asymptomatic stages)

matically infected with HIV[4]. In the United States, by June of 1989, over one million Americans were asymptomatically infected, with an annual incidence of approximately 40 000 new infections in American adolescents and adults[5].

Individuals who are asymptomatically infected with HIV remain infected, probably for life, and remain infectious. It is not known if HIV antibody positive individuals are infectious throughout the course of their infection. It may be that they are infectious (or more infectious) at different stages of the infection and non-infectious (or less infectious) at other stages. Infectivity may relate to the presence of HIV antigens in the blood.

It is currently not known how many individuals who are asymptomatically infected with HIV will eventually become ill. It may be, however, that over a twenty year period, most of them will develop some manifestation of ill health due to HIV acquisition. Considering the vast numbers of individuals now asymptomatically infected with this virus and the exponential rate of increase in this group, the magnitude of the epidemic becomes more sinister as the years go by. The chilling possibility of an entire generation of young people becoming ill, either with AIDS or with HIV-related neurological dysfunction, leaves little doubt that we are potentially facing the most serious threat to the public health in our human experience.

Phase B-2: Persistent generalized lymphadenopathy (PGL)

Many individuals infected with HIV develop a persistent, generalized lymphadenopathy (known as PGL or LAS – lymphadenopathy syndrome). PGL is defined as palpable lymph node enlargement (more than 1 cm) at two or more extra-inguinal sites for more than three months in the absence of an identifiable cause other than HIV infection. Axillary and cervical lymph nodes are commonly involved in this condition. Herpes (varicella) zoster commonly occurs in patients with PGL and may be a poor prognostic sign[6]. PGL can persist in some individuals for many years without any progression to clinical illness and it may be that this lymphadenopathy represents, in some individuals at any rate, a successful containment of the infection. However, it is now known that at least one third of patients with PGL develop AIDS over a five year period[7, 8]. This diagnostic term is generally reserved for those individuals in which lymphadenopathy is the principal manifestation of illness.

Phase C: The AIDS-related complex (ARC)

Many individuals develop a variety of indicators of ill health due to HIV infection *without developing major opportunistic infections or secondary cancers.* These constitutional symptoms and signs are sometimes referred to as the AIDS-related complex (ARC). Additionally, they may or may not have PGL. The diagnostic criteria for ARC are described in Table 5.2.

Additional laboratory findings in ARC would include a positive serology for antibodies to HIV.

Individuals with ARC usually appear chronically ill or even cachectic and may display a variety of minor opportunistic infections such as oral candidiasis (thrush) and skin conditions, for example seborrhoeic dermatitis. Seborrhoeic dermatitis presents as a red, scaly rash which commonly affects the face and scalp, although the entire body may be affected. This condition can occur in individuals with no prior history of skin disease and may be extremely serious. Some individuals also present with white, elevated lesions on the side of their tongue, known as hairy leucoplakia. Hairy leucoplakia is almost exclusively seen in patients with HIV infection and is thought to be caused by a virus (e.g. EBV or human papilloma virus)[9]. In addition, they are prone to a variety of bacterial, fungal and viral infections. *Tinea cruris* (a fungal

Table 5.2　Diagnostic criteria for ARC

The AIDS-related complex is diagnosed in a person who presents with any two or more signs/symptoms which have been present for three months or longer and any two or more abnormal laboratory values

Symptoms/signs
Fever: >38° C intermittent/continuous
Weight loss: >10%
Persistent generalized lymphadenopathy (PGL)
Diarrhoea: intermittent/continuous
Fatigue that reduces physical activity
Night sweats
Hairy leucoplakia
Oral candidiasis
Splenomegaly
Seborrhoeic dermatitis/folliculitis

Laboratory abnormalities
Lymphopenia, leucopenia ($<1.5 \times 10^9/1$)
Thrombocytopenia ($<150 \times 10^9/1$)
Anaemia
Reduced ratio of helper (T4) : suppressor (T8) cells ($>2SD$)
Reduced number of T4-helper cells ($<0.40 \times 10^9/1$)
Reduced blastogenesis
Raised serum levels of immunoglobulins
Cutaneous anergy to 3 recall antigens

skin disease of surfaces of contact in the scrotal, crural, and genital areas) and *Tinea pedis* (Athlete's foot) are frequently seen. Many individuals may also have enlarged spleens (splenomegaly) and most will have serological evidence of past exposure to various viruses, for example cytomegalovirus (CMV), Epstein-Barr virus (EBV), herpes simplex and hepatitis B virus. Herpes simplex infection may re-activate in patients with ARC and healing may be prolonged. Herpes zoster (shingles) infection may be seen in patients with ARC. Genital warts (*condyloma acuminata*) and molluscum contagiosum, presenting as large, multiple molluscum situated in the face, are sometimes seen in patients with ARC and both conditions are relatively unresponsive to conventional treatment. Testicular atrophy and malabsorptive diarrhoea are also seen and recently it has been reported that many patients with ARC develop unusually thick and elongated eyelashes[10].

Treatment is symptomatic.

Oral candidiasis – can be treated with topical antifungal preparations (e.g. nystatin or natamycin oral suspension) or if these fail, with systemic fluconazole.

Oral hairy leucoplakia – acyclovir ('Zovirax') or ganciclovir (DHPG) may be of some benefit[11].

Tinea cruris/pedis – treated with topical antifungal preparations such as 2% miconazole cream ('Daktarin') or 1% clotrimazole cream ('Canesten'), or with oral griseofulvin 125 mg four times daily.

Seborrhoeic dermatitis – treatment depends on location and severity. Tars are used to depress the proliferation of cells and have antipruritic and antiseptic properties. Salicylic acid is frequently combined with tars for its keratolytic action, i.e. helps remove scales allowing the tars access to the underlying diseased areas. Seborrhoeic dermatitis of the body can be treated with a combination of tars and salicylic acid, for example 'Gelcosal' and seborrhoeic dermatitis of the scalp can be treated with a similar preparation, for example 'Ionil T'. Topical steroids also reduce epidermal cell turnover and low-dose (0.5%) hydrocortisone cream can be used sparingly to treat small areas, the scalp and flexures. Aqueous creams are used and bath emollients (e.g. 'Aveeno Colloidal', 'Balneum', 'Alpha Keri') may be useful. 'Quinoderm Cream' (potassium hydroxyquinoline sulphate 0.5% with benzoyl peroxide 10%) is effective for facial folliculitis.

Herpes zoster – acyclovir ('Zovirax') is effective and is generally prescribed as 800 mg orally, five times a day (at four-hourly intervals) for seven days.

Herpes simplex – acyclovir ('Zovirax') is used and is generally prescribed as 200 mg orally, five times a day (at four-hourly intervals) for five days. Long-term, low-dose acyclovir prophylaxis may be required. Acyclovir-resistant lesions usually respond to trisodium phosphonoformate (Foscarnet) and sometimes to vidarabine.

Diarrhoea – antidiarrhoeals, for example loperamide hydrochloride ('Imodium'). diphenoxylate hydrochloride with atropine sulphate ('Lomotil') or codeine phosphate may be useful. If diarrhoea is severe, an oral fluid and electrolyte replacement preparation, such as 'Rehidrat' may be beneficial.

Malnutrition/cachexia – the patient should be assessed by a dietitian and an appropriate diet/dietary supplements implemented.

HIV infection – zidovudine ('Retrovir' – AZT) may be prescribed to treat the underlying cause.

Most patients with ARC will, in time (e.g. within 3 to 4 years), progress to fully expressed AIDS. Since the discovery of the causative agent of AIDS, and serological tests for detecting it, this diagnostic classification has become less useful. However as it is still widely used, it is included here.

Phase D: Major opportunistic infection(s) or secondary cancers, i.e. AIDS

The diagnosis of AIDS is made when Phase D first occurs.

AIDS

Patients are admitted to hospital for a variety of opportunistic infections associated with this syndrome. They are called 'opportunistic' as they are infections caused by pathogens which the body, in health, contains quite easily. However, in AIDS, these pathogens have taken the 'opportunity' of a depressed immune system to establish clinical illness. Although it is possible for a patient to be admitted with just one infectious disease, patients with AIDS more commonly present with a host of infections. We will look at each individually, remembering then that they frequently occur together in various combinations (Table 5.3).

Table 5.3 Opportunistic pathogens seen in HIV infection

Protozoal infections
  Pneumocystis carinii
  Toxoplasma gondii
  Cryptosporidium species
  Giardia lamblia
  Entamoeba histolytica
  Isospora species

Bacterial infections
  Mycobacterium tuberculosis
  Mycobacterium avium-intracellulare
  Mycobacterium kansasii/xenopi
  Salmonella typhimurium
  Shigella flexneri
  Legionella species
  Listeria monocytogenes
  Nocardia species

Fungal infections
  Candida albicans
  Cryptococcus neoformans
  Aspergillus species
  Coccidioides immitis
  Tinea species

Viral infections
  Cytomegalovirus
  Herpes simplex
  Herpes zoster
  Epstein-Barr virus
  Papovaviruses (JC/SV-40)

Pneumocystis carinii pneumonia (PCP)

PCP (also referred to as 'pneumocystosis') is not only the main present-ing disease seen in AIDS, it is by far the most frequent cause of death in persons with AIDS. The organism, first described in 1909 as a multi-flagellate protozoan and was first recognized as a human pathogen during World War II when it caused a fatal pneumonia in severely mal-nourished refugee children. P. Carinii is now thought to be a fungi, closely related to yeasts, rather than a protozoan[12]. *P. carinii* is part of the normal flora of most adults, rarely causing disease unless the immune system becomes compromised. In the United States, the first case of pneumonia in an adult caused by *P. carinii* was observed in 1954. Until the present epidemic of AIDS, PCP was only seen in patients whose immune system had been depressed by either a known primary or secondary cause, for example congenital immunodeficiency disorders, or patients receiving chemotherapy for cancer, or immuno-suppressant drugs following transplant surgery. It is a relatively important point for the nurse to note that PCP only occurs in immunocompromised individuals; hence hospital personnel and other patients, who are not immunocompromised, are not at risk of acquiring this infection.

Patients usually develop symptoms insidiously, often giving a three to four week history of cough, dyspnoea, chest pain, fever and chills. Tachypnoea (rapid respirations) and cyanosis are usually present when the patient is seen in hospital. Patients frequently complain of not being able to take a deep breath.

Some patients have a more fulminate course with a much shorter history. The patient may be in acute respiratory failure and in extreme distress.

The diagnosis of PCP is difficult. All the usual causes of pneumonia will need to be excluded and sputum will be obtained for routine culture and sensitivity. Chest X-rays usually show alveolar and interstitial infiltrates in both the right and left lung field (bilateral). These changes however, may be so mild as to be interpreted as normal in many patients. Abnormalities of arterial blood gases (associated with hypoxaemia) are common. The diagnosis of PCP is generally made as a result of bronchoalveolar lavage of subsegmental bronchi, or trans-bronchial biopsy, both distressing procedures in patients with an already established respiratory impairment. Biopsy can also help diagnose coexisting pulmonary infection with mycobacterium, CMV or *Cryptococcus neoformans*.

Nursing staff must wear protective clothing (a water-repellent, long-sleeved gown), disposable rubber latex or good quality plastic gloves, an effective, high filtration mask and eye protection when assisting with bronchoscopy.

A 'dedicated' bronchoscope is not necessary. Following bronchoscopy, the bronchoscope is thoroughly cleaned and then immersed in glutaraldehyde 2% for one hour. This is adequate disinfection and it can then be used for any other patient without fear of transmitting HIV[13].

Patients with PCP frequently have a dry, non-productive cough. The protocol for sputum induction consists of having the patient fast the night before sputum induction. To avoid contamination of the sputum specimen with oral debris, patients are asked to brush the buccal mucosa, tongue and gums with a wet toothbrush and rinse their mouths thoroughly with water. Sputum is then induced by inhalation of 20–30 ml of 3% saline through an ultransonic nebuliser. Gentle chest percussion to aid expectoration is used when necessary and two sputum specimens are then taken promptly to the laboratory. Examination of sputum obtained in this manner can detect evidence of Pneumocystis carinii infection in over 95% of patients, consequently sparing them from bronchoscopy[14]. Prior to sputum induction, chest x-rays are needed to rule out pleural effusions. Sputum induction is contraindicated in a patient with a pleural effusion as forceful coughing could fatally worsen the effusion[15].

Once PCP has been diagnosed, treatment is initiated with either pentamidine isethionate or trimethoprim-sulfamethoxazole ('Bactrim', 'Septrin').

Pentamidine isethionate – this drug is administered intravenously or intramuscularly in a dose of 4 mg/kg, once daily for at least 21 days.

Side-effects – almost half of all patients receiving pentamidine experience side-effects, ranging from nephrotoxicity (with elevated creatinine levels), hypoglycaemia (and sometimes, hyperglycaemia), sterile abscesses at the injection site, disorders of blood clotting (e.g. thrombocytopenia), skin rashes and pruritus (severe itching), tachycardia and hypotension. The abscesses at the injection site may become secondarily infected, providing yet another focus of infection for this immunocompromised patient and can be so painful that the patient may refuse further injections. Intramuscular injections into a wasted, catabolic patient present nursing care problems and although using alternative sites is helpful, the formation of abscesses, or the bleeding disorders sometimes caused by this drug, may preclude it being used intramuscularly.

For these reasons, intravenous administration of pentamidine is often preferred. Pentamidine, diluted in at least 250 ml of 5% dextrose/water, is given slowly (over 1–2 hours), once daily, under close supervision, as this route of administration has been associated with intractable hypotension.

Nursing implications of pentamidine therapy – urine specimens should be tested and blood glucose levels measured daily. Arterial blood pressure should be taken and recorded four-hourly, unless unstable, when it should be taken more frequently. During intravenous administrations of pentamidine, the blood pressure should be taken every 15 minutes.

Aerosolized Pentamidine The use of aerosolized pentamidine is also successful in both treating patients with PCP and as a prophylactic measure. Ultrasonic or jet nebulizers are used to deliver appropriate size particles of pentamidine (2–4 microns) into the alveoli. Pentamidine isethionate 600 mg. is dissolved in 6 ml of sterile water and shaken until all the solute is dissolved. The solution is stable for 48 hours at 20 degrees C. Using a 10 ml syringe, all the drug from the vial is withdrawn and injected into the drug chamber of the nebulizer system. The patient is treated in a sitting position and then lying on each side (to increase upper lobe distribution of the drug). The psi gas flow rate is determined by the nebulizer used but 6L/minute is usual. Aerosolized pentamidine should be administered in a room with good external ventilation and nursing personnel should wear effective, high filtration masks while caring for patients during this treatment[16]. The use of aerosolized pentamidine avoids many of the grave systemic side-effects of this drug. Side-effects of aerosolized pentamidine include cough and bronchospasm which can be treated with ipratropium bromide ('Atrovent'). Aerosolized pentamidine therapy can be used on an outpatient's basis and at home[17]. This form of treatment requires the use

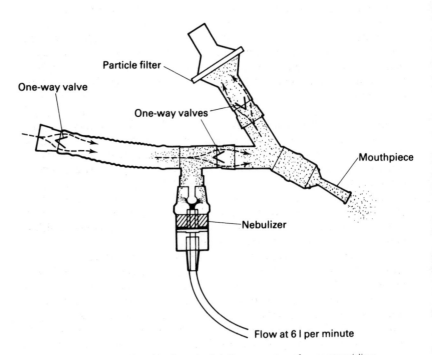

Fig. 5.2   Diagram of a nebulizer and delivery system for pentamidine aerosol

of a special nebulizer as shown in Fig. 5.2[18]. Extra-pumonary pneumosystis and pulmonary break-through infection with *P. carinii* can occur while clients are on prophylactic aerosolized pentamidine[19]. A nursing assessment for clients on such therapy must include a high index of suspicion for developing infections and their temperature must be taken at each visit.

Trimethoprim-sulfamethoxazole – also known as 'co-trimoxazole', is given in high doses (e.g. 20 mg trimethoprim/100 mg sulfamethoxazole/kg) either orally or intravenously, in divided doses, every eight hours, again for at least 21 days. Although generally this drug is associated with fewer side-effects than pentamidine, a high percentage of patients with AIDS (up to 80 per cent) develop a drug fever, rash and significant leucopenia when treated with this compound. Side-effects may be controlled by the administration of antihistamines, and/or by giving trimethoprim separately and reducing the dose of sulfonamide. Co-trimoxazole for intravenous use is diluted 1/25 in either 0.9% sodium chloride or 5% dextrose and is infused slowly (over one and a half hours) and care should be taken not to mistake *intramuscular* preparations for intravenous use. When given orally, nausea, vomiting and diarrhoea are not uncommon. It is usual for the medical staff to prescribe folinic acid (calcium folinate) 15 mg two to three times weekly in an attempt to prevent the bone marrow depression due to high dose trimethoprim-sulfamethoxazole therapy; this may be given orally or intravenously.

Other drugs used in the treatment of PCP include diaminodiphenylsulfone (Dapsone) with or without trimethoprim, DFMO (alpha difluromethylornithine), trimetrexate with leucovorin, the combination of clindamycin and primaquin or sulfadoxine and pyrimethamine (Fansidar).

All of these drugs have serious side effects and patients must be carefully observed for these, especially in the second week of therapy. The most common side effects include haematological abnormalities, nephrotoxicity and severe skin rashes.

Improvement, if it is to be seen, usually occurs within five to ten days. Although perhaps as many as 90 per cent of patients with AIDS who present with PCP can be successfully treated with the above drugs, they will eventually return to hospital with another episode, more difficult to treat. The long-term survival rate in patients, who have AIDS and present with PCP, is poor; the median cumulative survival is approximately 35 weeks. The quality of life is also poor with many patients (up to 40 per cent) spending more than half the time from date of diagnosis until death, in hospital.

Other causes of pneumonia in AIDS

The somewhat aggressive investigations required to diagnose PCP are needed, not only because the drugs used to treat this pneumonia are relatively toxic, hence the physician wants to be sure he actually is treating *P. carinii*, but also because several other opportunistic pathogens, some of which are treatable, are also known to cause pneumonia in patients with AIDS. These include mycobacteria (i.e. *M. tuberculosis* and atypical pneumonia caused by *M. avium intracellulare*, *M. xenopi*, *M. kansasii*), bacteria (e.g. *Streptococcus pneumoniae*, *Haemophilus influenzae*, *Pseudomonas aeruginosa*), viruses (e.g. CMV and herpes simplex), protozoa (e.g. *Toxoplasma gondii*) and fungi (*Aspergillus* and *Cryptococcus*). Most patients with Kaposi's sarcoma develop lung disease but it is usually asymptomatic. In some patients, KS may cause severe pulmonary symptoms (e.g. haemoptysis, dyspnoea, cough) and is unresponsive to treatment. Both lymphoid interstitial pneumonia and alveolar proteinosis are sometimes seen in patients with AIDS.

Mycobacterial infections are treated with anti-tuberculosis drugs such as rifampicin, ethambutol, isoniazid, and newer agents such as ansamycin and clofazimine. Bacterial infections are treated with the appropriate antibiotics as indicated by culture and sensitivity, and other therapies are available for some of the varied agents, which can cause pneumonia in the patient with AIDS. Bronchoalveolar lavage allows the physician to culture many of these opportunists and trans-bronchial biopsy (or open lung biopsy) can demonstrate pulmonary involvement of Kaposi's sarcoma.

Toxoplasmosis

Toxoplasmosis is caused by a small, intracellular protozoan parasite, *Toxoplasma gondii*. It exists as three forms (all potentially infectious to man) and is found in felines (cats) and some mammals. Man becomes infected when exposed to the parasite in cat faeces (e.g. litter trays or when gardening) or eating under-cooked infected beef, lamb or pork. Although man frequently becomes asymptomatically infected, it is only when the immune system fails to keep this parasite in check that it is able to cause clinical illness. In patients with AIDS, *T. gondii* can cause a variety of clinical disorders, but the most common illness seen related to infection with this agent is toxoplasma encephalitis.

Patients with toxoplasma encephalitis frequently present with neurological signs such as confusion, headache, vertigo and seizures. The patient often has an elevated temperature and is lethargic. The various signs and symptoms may resemble those seen in space-occupying lesions of the brain or those following stroke. The patient is seriously ill and can deteriorate with alarming speed.

Although encephalitis is by far the most frequent manifestation of toxoplasmosis in patients with AIDS, pneumonia and/or myocarditis can also occur.

In toxoplasma encephalitis, X-rays, CT scans, lumbar punctures and serological blood tests are usually abnormal, but changes seen are non-specific and the diagnosis is made by brain biopsy.

Once diagnosed, treatment is initiated with pyrimethamine and sulfadiazine. The usual doses used are: pyrimethamine – loading dose of 75 mg orally and then 25 mg orally, each day; sulfadiazine – 1g orally or intravenously, four times daily. Folinic acid (calcium folinate) 15 mg, in divided doses, daily, is often concurrently prescribed to prevent the serious consequences of depressed folate metabolism associated with pyrimethamine, for example leucopenia, thrombocytopenia and anaemia.

Intravenous clindamycin, with or without sulfadiazine or pyrimethamine may also be used. Newer macrolide antibiotices (e.g. azithromycin, roxithromycin) may also be used in the future. Corticosteroids and anticonvulsants may also be prescribed.

As it is impossible to eradicate *T. gondii* completely, treatment with these powerful drugs may have to continue for the remaining length of the patient's life.

Cryptosporidiosis

The protozoon, *Cryptosporidia*, has been recognized only in the last ten years as a potential human pathogen, causing a self-limited diarrhoea in animal workers (e.g. veterinarians and slaughterhouse workers). It is spread by a faecal-oral route and, in the immunodeficient individual, attacks the intestines (principally the small intestines), causing abdominal cramps, fever, nausea and vomiting and a profuse diarrhoea. In AIDS, this can be a catastrophic complication – diarrhoea can range from three to four bowel movements a day, to patients passing large amounts (10–12 litres/day) of watery diarrhoea, becoming hypotensive and showing signs and symptoms of electrolyte imbalance. This wasting, weakening disease attacks not only the small bowel, but also the patient's self-esteem, causing psychological havoc.

The diagnosis is made by using special techniques of staining smears of stool specimens or by biopsy of the gastrointestinal mucosa.

At the present time there is no specific therapy which is curative for this infection. Treatment with a macrolide antibiotic known as spiramycin ('Rovamycin' – May and Baker, 250 mg tablets) has been useful in some cases. It is given as one gram, 3–4 times daily for 1 to 16 weeks. Oral hyperimmune bovine colostrum has been used with limited success to treat this condition as has *Saccharomyces boulardii*[20].

Supportive treatment includes antidiarrhoeals, such as loperamide hydrochloride ('Imodium') and diphenoxylate hydrochloride with atropine sulphate ('Lomotil'), rehydration, electrolyte replacement, and nutritional support.

Diarrhoea is seen in most patients with AIDS and only in some is *Cryptosporidia* the cause. Other causes include amoebiasis (caused by the protozoon – *Entamoeba histolytica*) and giardiasis (caused by another protozoon, *Giardia lamblia*). These are not uncommon enteric infections in homosexuals and the diarrhoea seen is generally less than that seen in cryptosporidiosis. Amoebiasis is treated with oral metronidazole ('Flagyl') and di-iodohydroxyquin, and giardiasis is treated with atabrine or metronidazole.

Other opportunists associated with diarrhoea in patients with AIDS include *Shigella, Isospora belli, Helicobacter pylon* (*Campylobacter*), *Microsporidia, Salmonella, Strongyloides stercoralis, CMV,* and *Mycobacterium avium-intracellulare.* Kaposi's sarcoma may be an additional cause. Diarrhoea caused by isoporiasis is treated with co-trimoxazole ('Septrin', 'Bactrim') two tablets four times daily and metronidazole (e.g. 'Flagyl') is sometimes used to treat idiopathic diarrhoea. Diarrhoea is perhaps one of the most distressing complications of AIDS, and often one of the most difficult to treat.

Mycobacterial infections

There are several mycobacterial diseases associated with AIDS. The first one is *Mycobacterium avium-intracellulare* – a common potential pathogen that in the past rarely caused disease in man, even when immunocompromised. However, it is frequently seen as disseminated disease in patients with AIDS and presents as a disease similar to pulmonary tuberculosis. The disease then quickly disseminates to most organs in the body (spleen, bone marrow, lymph nodes, gastrointestinal tract, skin, and the brain), producing varied signs and symptoms, depending on which part of the body it was causing the most destruction. Patients generally have fever and chills, weight loss and fatigue.

Another mycobacterium sometimes associated with a lung condition similar to tuberculosis is *Mycobacterium kansasii*, which may also cause disseminated disease, cutaneous abscesses, bone and joint involvement, lymphadenitis and meningitis. Person-to-person transmission does not occur with either *M. avium-intracellulare* or *M. kansasii. Mycobacterium xenopi* can also cause pulmonary symptoms.

Mycobacterium tuberculosis causes pulmonary tuberculosis. Once the patient is immunocompromised, latent infections commonly flare up to produce active disease and as a result, pulmonary tuberculosis is seen in some patients with AIDS.

The diagnosis of mycobacterial infection involves biopsies of infected organs, chest X-rays and sputum cultures.

Although pulmonary tuberculosis usually can be controlled with routine anti-tuberculosis therapy, *Mycobacterium avium-intracellulare*, *M. xenopi* and *M. kansasii* are highly resistant to treatment. Various combinations of drugs may be tried, including clofazimine and ansamycin.

Cryptococcal infection

Infection caused by the fungus *Cryptococcus neoformans* (also known as *Filobasidiella neoformans*), a ubiquitous organism in nature, mainly causes meningitis in immunocompromised individuals. It can affect other areas in the body (e.g. lungs, bone, and the genito-urinary system) and prior to the current epidemic of AIDS was seen mainly in individuals with Hodgkin's disease.

Patients with AIDS may present with a slowly developing meningitis, complaining of headache, mild pyrexia and sometimes blurred vision. Other neurological signs and symptoms associated with meningitis (e.g. positive Kernig's sign, confusion, changes in level of consciousness) may develop, and the patient may become nauseated and start vomiting.

Cryptococcal meningitis is diagnosed by finding the fungus in cerebrospinal fluid, sputum, urine and blood cultures.

Drugs used for treating this severe infection include **amphotericin B**, **5-flucytosine** and fluconazole.

Amphotericin B ('Fungizone') is a major drug used to treat systemic fungal infections and is active against most fungi and yeasts. As it is frequently used for many of the systemic mycoses in patients with AIDS, it is covered in detail here. Amphotericin B is a fungicidal and fungistatic antibiotic and is given intravenously for systemic disease.

Amphotericin B is given in an initial dose of 0.25 mg/kg daily, increasing to 0.5 mg/kg daily to 1 mg/kg daily. The maximum daily dose is 1.5 mg/kg a day or on alternate days. Amphotericin B for intravenous infusion is available from pharmacy as a dry powder in a 50 mg vial. The vial must be kept refrigerated and protected from light. It is reconstituted with large volumes of 5% dextrose/water (*never* normal saline which can precipitate the drug) and is infused promptly after reconstitution via a central line over a six hour period. It is essential that the 5% dextrose infusion is issued by pharmacy and has a specific pH of greater than 4.2. Each container of 5% dextrose must be checked for its pH and the infusion container must be protected from light (the use of aluminum foil is convenient and effective) once the amphotericin has been added. Amphotericin B is a toxic drug and side-effects are common. Some patients experience chills, fever, headache, anorexia, nausea and occasionally vomiting, particularly with the initial infusion. Paracetamol (acetaminophen USP) and an antihistamine (e.g. chlorpheniramine maleate) may be prescribed concurrently with the infusion to lessen the incidence of these side-effects. Further side-effects include epigastric cramps, diarrhoea, haemorrhagic gastroenteritis with melaena, peripheral neuropathies, maculopapular rash, transient vertigo, tinnitus, hearing loss, blurred vision, diplopia, anaemia and convulsions. Rarely, anaphylactoid reactions, hypertension or hypotension, ventricular fibrillation and cardiac arrest can occur. Acute hepatic failure has also been encountered. Chemical thrombophlebitis may occur; adding 25 mg of hydrocortisone to the infusion may lessen the incidence—concomitant administration of heparin has not been shown to be helpful.[21] Serum potassium levels must be monitored frequently as hypokalaemia is common and occasionally is dramatic and dangerous. If hypokalaemia is detected, oral potassium supplements are usually adequate; if intravenous potassium is required, it is *not* added to the amphotericin B/5% dextrose solution. This drug is nephrotoxic and blood tests for renal function (e.g. blood urea nitrogen, serum creatinine) must be determined before and periodically during treatment. Patients must be monitored closely during therapy and vital signs are taken and recorded every 30 minutes during the infusion and for one hour after the infusion has completed. Corticosteroids may enhance the potassium depletion caused by amphotericin B. This potassium depletion may enhance the effects of curariform muscle relaxants and increase the toxicity of digitalis glycosides. It interacts with cyclosporin increasing the risk of nephrotoxicity.

It is possible to administer amphotericin B via an intrathecal injection. The usual technique employed for intrathecal injection is to first painstakingly dissolve 50 mg of amphotericin B in 10 ml of sterile water for injection. The total volume should then be diluted in a 250 ml bottle of 5% dextrose/water from which 10 ml has been removed. From 0.5 ml (0.1 mg) to 5.0 ml (1.0 mg) is then drawn into a 10 ml syringe, further diluted to 10 ml with CSF and injected *slowly* (over at least two minutes). A lumbar, cisternal, or ventricular (by an Ommaya reservoir) site may be used.

Flucytosine ('Alcobon') is available from the pharmacy department in a ready prepared 250 ml infusion (and administration set) containing 10 mg/ml. It is also available as 500 mg tablets. The usual dose by mouth or by intravenous infusion is 200 mg/kg daily in 4 divided doses. The dose is reduced in the presence of renal impairment. It is frequently given with amphotericin B for its synergistic effect on this drug. Flucytosine can cause nausea, vomiting, diarrhoea, rashes, thrombocytopenia and leucopenia. Weekly blood counts are necessary during prolonged treatment.

Fluconazole (Diflucan) is a novel triazole antifungal drug and may hopefully replace both amphotericin and flucytosine in the treatment of cryptococcal meningitis. It can be given either orally or intravenously; both routes are equally effective and it has a wide margin of safety and few side effects. It is given in a dose of 400 mg in a single dose on the first day, followed by a single daily dose of 200 mg. Intravenous fluconazole is supplied in either 25 ml or 100 ml bottles (each containing 2 mg. of fluconazole per ml). It is infused at a maximum rate of 200 mg. per hour as a continious infusion. Therapy with fluconazole usually continues for 10 to 12 weeks and CSF cultures become negative. For prophylaxis, the patient is continued on 100–200 mg. daily.

Viral infections – Herpesviruses

Patients with AIDS are particularly prone to infection with, or reactivation of, various herpesviruses, the most significant being cytomegaloviruses (CMV), herpes simplex viruses, varicella-zoster virus, and Epstein-Barr virus.

Cytomegalovirus infection

As children and young adults, most of us will have been exposed to **cytomegaloviruses** (CMV), a common, air-borne spread group of viruses ('salivary gland viruses'). CMV infection may also occur congenitally, postnatally, and can be acquired following blood transfusion ('Post-Perfusion Syndrome'). Infection with CMV produces variable results. Most infants infected show no clinical disease, but congenitally acquired CMV infection may cause abortion, stillbirth, postnatal death, or severe central nervous system damage. In children and adults who acquire this infection, most are asymptomatic, and a few may develop a mononucleosis or hepatitis. CMV are ubiquitous and 60–90 per cent of adults will have been exposed to this virus group and will have developed antibodies. When infected with CMV, individuals will excrete this virus in urine, saliva, cervical secretions, semen, faeces and breast milk for several months. Eventually, the process of cell-mediated immunity contains the infection, the individual developing a **latent infection**, and in most cases, never being aware that he or she had been infected in the first place. Like other latent infections normally contained by the immune system, in AIDS, CMV infection becomes re-activated as cell-mediated immunity is destroyed by HIV.

Most AIDS patients will have re-activated CMV infection and usually are viremic (i.e. have virus in their blood). In the constellation of opportunistic infections seen in patients with AIDS, it is often difficult to establish just what the clinical consequences of re-activated CMV infection are. However, as it may cause ulcerations of the gastro-intestinal tract, it may be implicated as yet another cause of diarrhoea seen in these patients. CMV can cause a terminal **pneumonitis** and also causes a **retinochoroiditis** which may lead to blindness.

Effective treatment for CMV infection has been unsatisfactory. New drugs currently being used are **ganciclovir (DHPG** – Syntex Corporation) and **trisodium phosphonoformate ('Foscarnet'** – Astra Pharmaceuticals). Ganciclovir 2.5–5 mg/kg is given intravenously every eight hours for 14–21 days. Patients with CMV pneumonitis and encephalitis do not respond well to ganciclovir and in CMV retino-pathy, it only seems to delay the progression of disease. Maintenance treatment (usually daily injections via a Hickman line) are usually necessary and these can be self-administered or administered by community nurses at home. Trisodium phosphonoformate 0.05–0.16 mg/kg per minute is administered by a continuous intra-venous infusion for 14–21 days, and is useful in ganciclovir-resistant infections.

The major side effect of Foscarnet therapy is nephrotoxicity and clients on this medication must be kept well hydrated. As ganciclovir (but not Foscarnet) may cause severe neutropenia, it is often not prescribed to individuals who are taking zidovudine (Retrovir – AZT). Clearly this may reduce its usefulness as most individuals who are at this stage of HIV disease will already be on zidovudine therapy. If both zidovudine and ganciclovir are being prescribed together, weekly white blood cell counts are usually done and nurses must be alert to developing pyogenic infections.

Herpes simplex virus infection

Many adults (including a large proportion of homosexual men) have been exposed to **herpes simplex** and consequently harbour these latent viruses. In AIDS they are frequently re-activated and may cause severe **perineal or facial lesions**. They will usually respond to treatment with the antiviral drug, **acyclovir**. Acyclovir-resistant lesions are usually treated with trisodium phosphonoformate (Foscarnate) or vidarabine.

Other viral infections

Many other latent viruses can be re-activated in AIDS and they include:

Varicella-zoster virus – causes herpes zoster (shingles) and is generally seen in patients with AIDS-related complex or PGL. Its occurrence may be prognostic of progression to fully expressed AIDS. These lesions respond to acyclovir, although oral acyclovir may have to be continued indefinitely to prevent relapse. This virus may also cause chickenpox (varicella) in non-immune individuals.

Epstein-Barr virus – may cause fever, lassitude and lymphadenopathy in patients with AIDS. There is no specific treatment available for illness associated with this virus.

Candidal species infection

Infection with **candidal species fungi** in healthy adults is now often associated as being a harbinger of AIDS. Most patients with AIDS have oral candidiasis ('thrush'), often affecting the oesophagus and rectum. Disseminated candidiasis can occur, but it is usually associated with indwelling catheters or prolonged treatment with antibiotics. Although sometimes responsive to treatment with nystatin or clotrimazole, candidiasis is frequently resistant to these agents. In such cases, fluconazole (Diflucan) is usually effective. Fluconazole is given orally as a single daily dose of 200 mg. on the first day, followed by 100 mg. daily. Candidal oesophagitis is serious and may cause perforation and haemorrhage. Treatment with the above agents, has to be continued for the remainder of the patient's life as, if discontinued, relapse is invariable.

Other opportunistic pathogens in AIDS

Although the opportunistic conditions we have discussed are the ones most frequently seen as a manifestation of immunodeficiency in patients with AIDS, and serve to define this disease, they are by no means the only potential pathogens which take the opportunity to establish clinical disease in the absence of immune competence. Other opportunists which may be encountered include:

Isospora belli – may cause severe diarrhoea.

Histoplasma capsulatum – causes **histoplasmosis**, a progressive, disseminating fungal disease involving lungs, spleen, liver and the gastro-intestinal tract.

Coccidioides immitis – causes **coccidioidomycosis**, another disseminated fungal disease involving many organs in the body including the brain, and may be involved in causing meningitis.

Nocardia asteroides – causes **nocardiosis**, a disseminating disease associated with metastatic brain abscesses, skin or subcutaneous abscesses and pulmonary lesions.

Listeria monocytogenes – causes **listeriosis**, meningitis being its most frequent clinical presentation.

Papova viruses – JC virus and SV-40 virus have been implicated in causing a severe, progressive, demyelinating disease in patients with AIDS, known as **progressive multifocal leucoencephalopathy (PML)**. This is a rare but serious infection of the central nervous system for which there is no effective therapy at present.

Salmonella – these Gram-negative bacteria commonly cause an enteritis from which septicaemia (*salmonellosis*) frequently develops in patients with AIDS. Drugs used to treat this condition include ampicillin, amoxicillin or chloramphenicol. The septicaemia is recurrent and often unresponsive to treatment[21].

Shigella – These are also Gram-negative bacteria and, like *Salmonella*, belong to a family of bacteria known as Enterobacteriaceae. *Shigella* cause enteritis, dysentery and like *Salmonella*, can cause a persistent bacteraemia in patients with AIDS. Drugs used to treat this condition include ampicillin, tetracycline and co-trimoxazole.

All patients with AIDS will develop opportunistic infection at some time during the course of their illness. Even though most are initially treatable, eventually they become more difficult, if not impossible, to treat and eventually, after incapacitating illness, cause death in patients with AIDS.

The other remaining major opportunistic disease seen in AIDS is Kaposi's sarcoma.

Kaposi's sarcoma

Prior to the current epidemic of AIDS, Kaposi's sarcoma (KS) was a relatively unusual vascular tumour, first described by a Hungarian dermatologist, Moriz Kaposi, in 1872. In the United States and in Western Europe, Kaposi's sarcoma was mainly seen in elderly men, especially those of Italian or Eastern European Jewish ancestry, and was relatively benign in its clinical course. Patients presented with discoloured patches, plaques, or nodular skin lesions, brown, red or blue in colour, usually confined to lower extremities (especially the ankles and soles of the feet). These lesions are the result of a multicentric tumour arising from local hyperplasia of a cell of the vascular endothelium. Often, as the patients were in the age group 60–79 years, no specific treatment was indicated. This type of indolent, non-aggressive, non-invasive Kaposi's sarcoma has become known as **classic** Kaposi's sarcoma.

Another form of Kaposi's sarcoma was known to exist in Equatorial Africa, where it was more common. Four different types of Kaposi's sarcoma have been described in Africa, one of which is similar to classic Kaposi's sarcoma, the remaining three being more aggressive, rapidly progressive neoplastic conditions, affecting young African men, often fatal within a year. This African form of Kaposi's sarcoma is sometimes referred to as **endemic** Kaposi's sarcoma.

Prior to 1981, a type of Kaposi's sarcoma similar to the African endemic form was observed in renal patients following kidney transplant and iatrogenic immunosuppression. This too was aggressive, but responded well to discontinuation of immunosuppression therapy and restoration of the patient to immune competence.

With the advent of AIDS in 1981, an aggressive form of Kaposi's sarcoma, similar to African endemic Kaposi's sarcoma, was seen in young, previously healthy male homosexuals. This AIDS-associated Kaposi's sarcoma has become known as **epidemic** Kaposi's sarcoma and patients usually present with asymptomatic, pigmented skin lesions which may be on any part of the body. Lesions can usually be identified in the mouth, especially on the hard palate, and many will also have lymph node enlargement. The initial lesions are often multifocal at time of diagnosis, often involving visceral organs (e.g. lungs, liver, spleen, gastrointestinal tract), and rapidly disseminate, usually in an orderly fashion.

The average life expectancy of patients with AIDS who have Kaposi's sarcoma is about 16 months, only a quarter of all patients surviving for two years or more.

Treatment does not improve survival, or the rate of the appearance of new lesions. However, it is useful for palliation and various treatment modalities can be effectively used.

Local irradiation therapy – skin and oral lesions are often radiosensitive and doses under 20 Gy are used.

Interlesional chemotherapy – small cutaneous lesions are sometimes treated for cosmetic purposes with interlesional injections of 0.01 mg of vinblastine in 0.1 ml of sterile water, using a tuberculin syringe. This has to be frequently repeated and a hyperpigmented area frequently remains following treatment.

Systemic Chemotherapy – various anti-cancer drugs have been tried and currently the following have been found to be the most useful. **Vinblastine** (given intravenously, once weekly in doses of 4–10 mg). This regime is associated with minimal toxicity and approximately 40 per cent of patients treated may show objective improvement. **VP-16 (epidophyllotoxin)** (given intravenously for 3 days every 3–4 weeks in doses of 150 mg per square metre of body surface). Most patients will experience side-effects, especially leucopenia and alopecia; however up to 75 per cent may show objective improvement.

One of the dangers of anti-cancer chemotherapy is the risk of further depressing the immune system and rendering the patient more prone to opportunistic infection. The use of VP-16 is not only associated with the highest objective response rate, but is also associated with the lowest rate of occurrence of opportunistic infection (seen in only 12 per cent of patients treated, as opposed to 25 per cent of patients treated with vinblastine).

Immune modulators – it seemed clear from the beginning of the epidemic that curative treatment for epidemic Kaposi's sarcoma would be available only if immune competence was restored, and various immune modulators have been used in combination with anti-cancer chemotherapy. **Alpha-interferons** have been widely used to stimulate the immune system in patients with AIDS and may be useful in treating epidemic Kaposi's sarcoma. However this has not been shown to restore immune competence. Intravenous administration has been shown to be associated with the fewest side-effects, which commonly include fever, malaise, headache, and transient, mild confusion. Alpha-interferon is often combined with zidovudine (Retrovir – AZT) as they exhibit synergistic activity in this disease.

Other tumours in AIDS

Although Kaposi's sarcoma is by far the most common malignancy seen in AIDS, **undifferentiated lymphomas** (non-Hodgkin's lymphomas), affecting various sites including the central nervous system, bone marrow and gastrointestinal tract, may be seen. An increased incidence of other tumours may also be encountered. It may be that the various viruses present in patients with AIDS, or infected with HIV are potentially oncogenic and once the immune system has broken down, may become involved in the pathogenesis of the various tumours seen.

Phase E: Periods of remission

Treatment of the opportunistic diseases encountered in AIDS will produce periods of remission and relative good health. This phase of AIDS can be considerably prolonged if the patient is commenced on zidovudine therapy. However, neurological dysfunction from either CNS opportunistic disease secondary to HIV infection, or to the direct action of HIV on nervous tissues (e.g. dementia) may seriously limit the relative health of patients with AIDS who are in remission. Periods of remission alternate with new opportunistic diseases (i.e. Phase D) and eventually, patients proceed to Phase F.

Phase F: Terminal phase of illness

Patients eventually develop terminal opportunistic illnesses from which they will die. Pneumonia caused by *Pneumocystis carinii* is the most common cause of death in patients with AIDS. In this phase, patients are frequently blind (due to CMV retinitis), bed-bound and incontinent, dementing and grossly malnourished and wasted. They may be extremely frightened and only nursing care of the highest quality is able to make a critical impact on the physical and psychological condition of these young patients who find themselves wide awake in their own worst nightmare.

Classification system for HIV infection

In 1986, the Centers for Disease Control (CDC) outlined a system which classified the manifestations of HIV infection into four mutually exclusive groups, designated by Roman numerals I through IV (Table 5.4)[22]. Classification in a particular group is not explicitly intended to have prognositic significance, nor to designate severity of illness. However, classification in the four principal groups, I–IV, is hierarchical in that persons classified in a particular group should not be reclassified in a preceding group if clinical findings resolve, since clinical improvements may not accurately reflect changes in the severity of the underlying disease.

Group I – this refers to the acute seroconversion illness described in Phase A (p. 38).

Group II – this refers to asymptomatic HIV infection described in Phase B-1 (pp. 38–39).

Table 5.4   Summary of classification system for HIV infection

Group I	Acute infection
Group II	Asymptomatic infection
Group III	Persistent generalized lymphadenopathy
Group IV	Other diseases
Subgroup A	Constitutional disease
Subgroup B	Neurological disease
Subgroup C	Secondary infectious diseases
Category C-1	Specified secondary infectious diseases listed in the CDC surveillance definition for AIDS
Category C-2	Other specified secondary infectious diseases
Subgroup D	Secondary cancers
Subgroup E	Other conditions

Group III – this refers to PGL as described in Phase B–2 (p. 39).

Group IV – other HIV diseases: the clinical manifestations of patients in this group may be designated by assignment to one or more subgroups (A–E) listed below.

Subgroup A – this refers to patients previously classified as having the AIDS-related complex (ARC), i.e. Phase C (pp. 39–42).

Subgroup B – this refers to patients who develop neurological manifestations of HIV infection, i.e. Phase D (pp. 42–59).

Subgroup C – this is defined as the diagnosis of an infectious disease associated with HIV infection and/or at least moderately indicative of a defect in cell-mediated immunity. Patients in this subgroup are divided further into two categories:

Category C-1 includes patients with symptomatic or invasive disease due to one of the specified secondary infectious diseases listed in the surveillance definition of AIDS (Appendix 1), i.e. Phase D.

Category C-2 includes patients with symptomatic or invasive disease due to one of six specified secondary infectious diseases: oral hairy leucoplakia, multidermatomal herpes zoster, recurrent *Salmonella* bacteraemia, nocardiosis, tuberculosis, or oral candidiasis, i.e. can be either Phase C or Phase D.

Subgroup D – defined as the diagnosis of one or more kinds of cancer known to be associated with HIV infection as listed in the surveillance definition of AIDS (Appendix 1), i.e. Phase D.

Subgroup E – defined as the presence of other clinical findings or diseases, not classifiable above, that may be attributed to HIV infection and/or may be indicative of a defect in cell-mediated immunity. Included are patients with adult chronic lymphoid interstitial pneumonitis. Also included are those patients whose signs or symptoms could be attributed either to HIV infection or to another coexisting disease not classified elsewhere, and patients with other clinical illnesses, the course or management of which may be complicated or altered by HIV infection. Examples include: patients with constitutional symptoms not meeting the criteria for subgroup IV-A; patients with infectious diseases not listed in subgroup IV–C; and patients with neoplasms not listed in subgroup D.

This classification system is meant to provide a means of grouping patients infected with HIV according to the clinical expression of disease. It defines a limited number of specified clinical presentations.

WHO Clinical Staging System for HIV Infection and Disease

In 1990, the World Health Organisation drafted a staging system for HIV infection and disease, which is reproduced in **Appendix 2**.

Summary

Fully expressed AIDS is an acquired immunodeficiency state in which individuals develop one or more opportunistic infections, usually due to latent, potential pathogens which are ubiquitous in nature and which, were it not for the underlying immune deficiency, would not be dangerous. The most common opportunistic infection seen is pneumonia, caused by the fungi, *Pneumocystis carinii*. The depressed immune state also involves a breakdown in the normal tumour surveillance carried out by activated natural killer cells and opportunistic cancers may be seen, chiefly Kaposi's sarcoma.

Treatment for either opportunistic infectious diseases or cancers is not curative as the principal defect is in the immune system and, until a way can be found to restore the competence of this system, AIDS will continue to be a fatal disease.

References

1.   Centers for Disease Control (1987). Revision of the CDC Surveillance Case Definition for Acquired Immunodeficiency Syndrome. *MMWR* (August 14), 36:1S

2.   Mildvan, D. and Solomon, S.L. (1987). The spectrum of disease due to Human Immunodeficiency Virus Infection, in *Current Topics in AIDS Volume 1*, ed. by Gottlieb, M., Jeffries, D., and Mildvan, D., *et al.* p 35. John Wiley & Sons, UK

3.   *Ibid.*

4.   PHLS Communicable Disease Surveillance Centre (1990). Acquired Immune Deficiency Syndrome in England and Wales to End of 1993 – Projections using data to end September 1989: Report of a Working Group ('The Day Report'), *Communicable Disease Report* (January), UK

5.   Centers for Disease Control (1990). Estimates of HIV Prevalence and Projected AIDS Cases: Summary of a Workshop, October 31–November 1, 1989, *MMWR*, 39(7):110–119

6.   Weber, J., Pinching, A. (1986). The clinical management of AIDS and HTLV–III Infection, in *The Management of AIDS Patients*, ed. by Miller, D., Weber, J., and Green, J. p 11. The Macmillan Press Ltd, London

7.   Mathur-Wagh, U., Mildvan, D., Van Camp, J., *et al.* (1986). Persistent generalized lymphadenopathy (PGL) in homosexual men: a comparison of two cohorts. *Program and Abstracts of the Second International Conference on AIDS.* Paris, June 1986:115

8.   Metroka, C.E., Cunningham-Rundles, S., Krim, M., *et al.* (1986). A four year perspective study of clinical and immunological parameters of patients with generalized lymphadenopathy. *Program and Abstracts of the Second International Conference on AIDS.* Paris, June 1986:123

9.   Mindel, A. (1987). Management of early HIV Infection, in *ABC of AIDS*, ed. by Adler, M.W. p. 16. British Medical Journal, London

10. Mildvan, D. and Solomon, S.L. (1987). *op. cit.* p 37

11. Newman, C., Polk, B.F. (1987). Resolution of oral hairy leucoplakia during therapy with 9-(1,3-dihydroxy-2-proproxymethyl) guanine (DHPG). *Annals of Internal Medicine*, 107(3):348–350

12. Edman, J.C., Kovacs, J.A., Masur, H., *et al.* (1988). Ribosomal RNA sequence shows Pneumocystis carinii to be a member of the fungi, *Nature* 334(5):19

13. UK Health Departments (1990). *Guidance for Clinical Health Care Workers: Protection Against Infection with HIV and Hepatitis Viruses, Recommendations of the Expert Advisory Group on AIDS*, p 40, HMSO, London

14. Leigh, T.R., Parsons, P., Hume, C., *et al.* (1989). Sputum Induction For Diagnosis of Pneumocystis Carinii Pneumonia, *Lancet* (July 22). ii(8656):205–206

15. Nelson, M., Bower, M., Smith, D., Gazzard, B.G. (1990). Life-threatening complication of sputum induction (correspondence), *Lancet* (January 13), 335:112–113

16. Smith, C.L. (1990). Nursing Management of Aerosolized Pentamidine Administration, *AIDS Patient Care* (February) 4(1):13–17

17. Green, S.T., Nathwani, D., Christie, P.R., *et al.*, (1990). Domicilliary nebulized pentamidine for secondary prophylaxis against Pneumocystis

carinii pneumonia, *Journal of the Royal Society of Medicine*, **83**(1):18–19
18. Montgomery, A.B., Luce, J.M., Turner, J. *et al.* (1987). Aerosolised Pentamidine as sole therapy for Pneumocystis carinii pneumonia in patients with Acquired Immunodeficiency Syndrome, *Lancet* (August 29), **ii**(8557):480–82
19. Northfeldt, D.W. (1989). Extrapulmonary pneumocystosis in patients taking aerosolised pentamidine, *Lancet* (December 16) **ii**, London
20. Saint-Marc, T., Sellem, C., Rosello, L., *et al.* (1990). Treatment of Chronic Diarrhoea with *Saccharomyces baulardii*, VI International Conference on AIDS (San Francisco), *Abstracts*, Th. B. 363.
21. Panther, L.A., Sande, M.A. (1990). Cryptococcal Meningitis in AIDS, in *The Medical Management of AIDS*, (ed.) Sande, M.A. and Volberding, P.A., 2nd ed., p 273, W.B. Saunders Co., London
22. Centers for Disease Control (1986). Classification System for Human T-Lymphotropic Virus Type III/Lymphadenopathy-Associated Virus Infection. *MMWR* (May 23), **35**(20):334–39

Further reading

Sande, M.A. and Volberding, P.A. (1990). *The Medical Management of AIDS*, 2nd ed., W.B. Saunders Co., London
Levy, J.A. (1989). *AIDS – Pathogenesis and Treatment*, Marcel Dekker, Inc., New York and Basel

6

Caring for Patients with Neuropsychiatric Manifestations of HIV Infection

It is now well established that HIV acquisition is frequently associated with a variety of neuropsychiatric syndromes[1]. Neuropsychiatric syndromes refer to both central nervous system (CNS) diseases and organic mental disorders and may be due to opportunistic infections, neoplastic processes or the primary effect that HIV has on the CNS. In assessing and planning care, it is essential that the nurse has a sound knowledge of the potential neurological consequences of HIV infection. Neuropsychiatric manifestations of HIV infection include those described in Table 6.1.

Neurological dysfunction may be the first manifestation of HIV infection. Early neurological syndromes include atypical aseptic meningitis, acute encephalitis and acute peripheral neuropathy. These syndromes may appear soon after HIV infection at the time of seroconversion.

Atypical aseptic meningitis

Aseptic meningitis is a febrile meningeal inflammation due to early CNS infection with HIV.

Patients frequently seek medical advice because of various meningeal signs (Table 6.2). This type of aseptic meningitis (**aseptic** being the term

Table 6.1 Neuropsychiatric manifestations of HIV infection

Atypical aseptic meningitis	
Acute encephalitis	
Peripheral neuropathy	
Autonomic neuropathy	
Vacuolar myelopathy	Due to neurotrophic effects of HIV
Landry-Guillain-Barré syndrome	
Subclinical cognitive dysfunction	
Organic mental disorders	
CNS opportunistic infections	
CNS neoplastic disease	
Cerebrovascular disorders	

Table 6.2   Meningeal signs

Fever
Drowsiness
Stiff neck
Headache
Vomiting

applied to meningitis caused by viruses and other pathogens without any evidence of bacterial organisms in the CSF) is complicated by additional features (i.e. **atypical**) not generally seen in patients with aseptic meningitis. These atypical features include cranial nerve dysfunction, especially involvement of cranial nerves V, VII and VIII[2]. Involvement of the trigeminal (V) and facial (VII) nerves may evoke facial numbness, palsy and paralysis and trigeminal neuralgia. Involvement of the auditory (VIII) nerve may produce tinnitus, deafness and vertigo. Other atypical features include the tendency for this type of meningitis to recur and to become chronic.

Investigations include lumbar puncture and head CT (computerized tomography) scanning. A CT scan is desirable in patients in which HIV infection is being considered to exclude intracerebral abscess caused by *Toxoplasma gondii*, which may present in a similar fashion. Lumbar puncture then might be contraindicated due to the risk of a change in the CSF pressure, caused by the sudden withdrawal of fluid from the spinal canal, precipitating herniation of the medulla and cerebellar tonsils into the foramen magnum (i.e. **coning**) with fatal results.

CSF obtained from lumbar puncture usually shows a normal glucose level (50–100 mg/100 ml), a normal or only slightly elevated protein content (20–45 mg/100 ml), an increase in mononuclear or polymorphonuclear white cells, lymphocytic pleocytosis (i.e. an excessive number of lymphocytes in the CSF) and the absence of bacterial growth on culture. HIV has been detected in the CSF in patients with atypical aseptic meningitis[3].

Atypical aseptic meningitis may be either acute or chronic and, in general, complete recovery can be expected. Medical treatment is entirely symptomatic (e.g. analgesics and antipyretics), although zidovudine (Retrovir – AZT) may be used. Fluid balance is maintained but care is taken not to overhydrate the patient.

Acute encephalitis

Acute encephalitis is an acute inflammatory disease of the brain due to direct HIV invasion and/or hypersensitivity initiated by HIV infection

Table 6.3   Acute encephalitis – signs of cerebral dysfunction

Alterations in level of consciousness
Personality change
Seizures
Paresis
Focal neurological signs

of the brain. Like acute atypical meningitis, acute encephalitis occurs most frequently soon after HIV infection, at the time of seroconversion[4]. Acute encephalitis differs from atypical aseptic meningitis in that there is evidence of cerebral dysfunction (Table 6.3), which is independent of signs of meningeal inflammation.

Investigations include a CT scan and lumbar puncture to exclude cryptococcal meningitis and intracerebral abscess caused by *Toxoplasma gondii*. Acute encephalitis is a more serious condition than atypical aseptic meningitis and, although recovery can be expected, high-dependency nursing care is required to maintain a safe environment for the patient to recover. The patient's need for nutrition, adequate hydration and to maintain a normal body temperature, must be carefully assessed and facilitated. Antipyretics and anticonvulsant medications may be prescribed and zidovudine (Retrovir – AZT) may be used. Both atypical aseptic meningitis and acute encephalitis are medical emergencies and patients must be admitted to hospital for immediate treatment and to assist the patient to meet his safety needs.

Peripheral neuropathy

HIV infection of peripheral nerves (e.g. cranial and spinal nerve) may cause symptoms either prior to or after the development of ARC or fully expressed AIDS (often seen in patients with subacute encephalitis). Peripheral neuropathy may be either acute, subacute or chronic.

There is symmetrical involvement of both sensory and motor nerves (i.e. **symmetrical sensorimotor neuropathy**) and patients frequently complain of the occurrence of spontaneous pains (**dysaesthesia**) and pain which is provoked by gentle, light touch or temperature stimulation (**hyperaesthesia**).

There may be weakness and wasting in the arms and legs (i.e. **distal atrophy**). Involvement of the spinal nerve roots may produce pain referred to the back of the thigh and leg below the knee, weakness, flaccidity and eventually atrophy of the legs (**radicular syndrome**).

Involvement of a peripheral nerve on one side of the body

(**asymmetric**) is characterized by a sensation of numbness, prickling or tingling (i.e. **paraesthesia**), pain and weakness. This condition is known as 'mononeuritis multiplex' and may present prior to the development of AIDS.

Acute peripheral neuropathy may present as a facial paralysis and involve only one side of the face ('Bell's palsy').

Zidovudine (Retrovir – AZT) may be used to treat this condition.

Vacuolar myelopathy

HIV frequently has a direct effect on both motor and sensory nerves in the spinal cord in patients with AIDS and produces a paraesthesia, weakness and spasticity of the legs. There may be a failure or irregularity of muscular coordination, especially manifested when voluntary muscular movements are attempted (ataxia). Urinary incontinence may develop. This condition is known as vacuolar myelopathy and may be seen in patients with subacute encephalitis. Zidovudine (Retrovir – AZT) may be used to treat this condition.

Autonomic neuropathy

Damage to the autonomic nervous system can result in erectile failure, some cases of unexplained diarrhoea or cardiovascular instability. The latter may lead to postural hypotension, fainting and cardiovascular arrest. Erectile failure may be treated with alpha-adrenoceptor blocking agents such as **yohimbine**. Diarrhoea due to autonomic neuropathy may respond to treatment with adrenergic neurone blocking drugs such as **guanethidine** ('Ismelin'). Hypotension associated with autonomic neuropathy may be effectively treated with **fludrocortisone** ('Florinef').

Other neurological syndromes

Landry-Guillain-Barré syndrome. This is an acute, rapidly progressive form of polyneuropathy characterized by muscular weakness and various disorders of movement, due to involvement of the spinal roots and peripheral nerves, which may also be seen in patients with AIDS[5].

Subclinical cognitive dysfunction. Most patients with AIDS, without known neurological complications, will develop impairment of reasoning, perception, intuition, memory, language and ability to learn. This is probably due to diffuse cerebral dysfunction of the dominant hemisphere[6].

Organic mental disorders

Organic mental disorders (OMD) are extremely common in patients with AIDS, being seen in upwards of 70 per cent of all patients. They are classified as being either acute or chronic[7].

Acute organic mental disorders

Delirium is the major acute OMD seen in patients with AIDS and is characterized by an altered and/or fluctuating level of consciousness. Delirium has an acute onset, is secondary to underlying conditions seen in patients with AIDS (Table 6.4) and, typically, resolves completely within a week without any ill effects.

Treatment is aimed at correcting the underlying cause and maintaining a safe environment for the patient during this period. Sedatives and analgesics should not be given during this episode as they further depress the cerebral cortex.

Table 6.4   Causes of acute OMD in patients with AIDS

CNS opportunistic infections
Meningitis (e.g. atypical aseptic meningitis)
HIV encephalopathy
CNS neoplasms
Seizure disorders and post-seizure states
Septicaemia
Cerebral hypoxia
Electrolyte imbalance (e.g. hyponitraemia, hypokalaemia, hyper- or
   hypoglycaemia)
Cerebral oedema
Cerebrovascular infarction or haemorrhage
Pyrexia
Brain abscess
Environmental factors (e.g. isolation, distress, sleep deprivation)
Drugs (side-effects) and alcohol

Chronic organic mental disorders

Chronic organic mental disorders are more frequently encountered in individuals infected with HIV than acute OMD[8]. **Dementia** is the predominant chronic OMD seen in patients with AIDS and, like acute OMD, has a multifactorial aetiology (Table 6.5).

Table 6.5   Causes of chronic OMD in patients with AIDS

HIV encephalopathy
Progressive encephalitis due to other viruses (e.g. CMV, herpes simplex,
   varicella zoster and JC virus)
Space-occupying lesions caused by B cell lymphoma or (rarely) Kaposi's
   sarcoma
Space-occupying lesions caused by infectious agents (e.g. *Candida
   albicans, Toxoplasma gondii, Cryptococcus neoformans*)
Cerebrovascular accidents

The most common cause of dementia is the direct effect of HIV
infection on either cerebral cortical or subcortical structures of the
brain. This is referred to as **HIV encephalopathy** (AIDS dementia
Complex, or ADC).

Dementia due to HIV encephalopathy has an insidious onset. There
is a progressive loss of cognitive function, beginning with problems
coping with complicated tasks and ending with a bed-bound, incontinent individual. A careful nursing assessment will reveal various
indicators of cortical dysfunction as described in Table 6.6. The clinical
staging of HIV encephalopathy is described in Table 6.7.

The objective of medical management is to treat the underlying

Table 6.6   HIV encephalopathy: indicators of cortical dysfunction

---

1. Disorders of intellect
    (a) Memory loss
    (b) Short attention span and impairment in ability to concentrate
    (c) Deterioration in learning abilities and ability to abstract
    (d) Slow and difficult thinking
    (e) Blunting of perception and errors of judgement

2. Disorders of behaviour
    (a) Social withdrawal
    (b) Disinhibited or embarrassing and anti-social behaviour
    (c) Deterioration in self-care (e.g. lack of attention to personal
        cleanliness, dress and nutrition)

3. Disorders of mood
    (a) Labile emotions (easily frustrated, irritable, quickly changing mood)
    (b) Anxiety
    (c) Depression

4. Disorders of personality
    (a) Former personality traits accentuated
    (b) Interpersonal relationships altered
    (c) Demanding behaviour and egocentricity

Table 6.7　Clinical staging of HIV encephalopathy

Stage	Characteristics
Stage 0 (Normal)	Normal mental and motor function
Stage 0.5 (equivocal/ subclinical)	Either minimal or equivocal evidence of motor impairment; can work and perform activities of daily living
Stage 1.0 (mild)	Unequivocal evidence of functional impairment; able to do all but demanding tasks
Stage 2.0 (moderate)	Cannot work but can perform basic activities of self care
Stage 3.0 (severe)	Major intellectual incapacity or motor disability
Stage 4.0 (end stage)	Nearly vegatative

cause. Zidovudine (Retrovir – AZT) may produce significant improvement in patients with HIV encephalopathy.

Opportunistic infections of the CNS

Opportunistic CNS infections account for many of the neurological syndromes seen in individuals with AIDS. The most frequent causes of opportunistic CNS infections in patients with AIDS are shown in Table 6.8.

Table 6.8　CNS opportunistic infections in patients with AIDS

Toxoplasma gondii
Cryptococcus neoformans
Herpes simplex
Cytomegalovirus
Candida albicans
Mycobacterium tuberculosis
Mycobacterium avium-intracellulare
Papovavirus

Toxoplasma gondii

Intracerebral abscess caused by the protozoon *Toxoplasma gondii* is one of the most common opportunistic CNS infections seen in patients with AIDS. It is manifested by an insidious onset of confusion and lethargy prior to the development of focal neurological deficits (e.g. seizures) or a diminished level of consciousness. The clinical diagnosis is confirmed by head computerized tomography (CT) scans, magnetic resonance imaging (MRI) scans and lumbar puncture. CT scans frequently demonstrate cerebral ring-enhancing lesions and magnetic resonance imaging scans may be positive. CNS fluid from lumbar punctures may show an increased concentration of protein (i.e. more than 20–45 mg/100 ml) and it may be possible to isolate the organism from the CSF[9]. However, lumbar puncture may be contraindicated due to the risk of 'coning'.

A toxoplasma serology (indirect immunofluorescence assay or Sabin-Feldmann dye inclusion test) may be positive and a brain biopsy may be required to confirm the diagnosis. Treatment of CNS toxoplasma infection incorporates the use of **pyrimethamine** and **sulfadiazine**. **Clindamycin, spiramycin** and **sulfadoxine** may also be used[10]. **Dexamethasone** or **mannitol** and/or diuretics are given if there is cerebral oedema. Maintenance treatment is required for the rest of the patient's life as relapse after cessation of treatment is common. **Maloprim**, a combination of **Dapsone** (a bacteriostatic sulphone) and **pyrimethamine**, is commonly used for maintenance therapy. Toxoplasma infection of the CNS is associated with a high mortality in patients with AIDS. Toxoplasma may also cause visual dysfunction (chorioretinitis).

Cryptococcus neoformans

A granulomatous meningitis, with granulomas or cysts developing in the cerebral hemispheres, typically results from cryptococcal fungal infection of the CNS. Patients present with a history of headache, high fever, nausea and vomiting and photophobia. Some may also experience seizures. CNS fluid from lumbar puncture may be normal or show an increased number of cells (pleocytosis), increased protein and a lowered glucose content (i.e. less than 50–100 mg/100 ml). CT scans are usually normal, although they may show hydrocephalus and/or cerebral atrophy. The diagnosis is confirmed by indian ink staining of CSF fluid, cultures of CSF or the detection of cryptococcal antigens in CSF fluid or serum.

Medical treatment consists of **amphotericin B** and **5-flucytosine** by intravenous infusion through a central line. Amphotericin B has significant side-effects, which include rigors, fever and renal damage (e.g. hypokalaemia). Antihistamine cover with **chlorpheniramine maleate** ('Piriton') is common while patients are being treated with amphotericin B. Relapse is common and can be predicted by a rise in serum cryptococcal antigen titre. Therefore, monthly maintenance treatment (with the same drugs via a peripheral line) for the rest of the patients' life is usual. **Fluconazole** (Diflucan) is now replacing amphotericin B and 5-flucytosine as the treatment of choice for crypto-coccal meningitis as it can be given either orally or intravenously and has few side effects. Therapy with fluconazole is initiated with a single dose of 400 mg. (either orally or intravenously) on the first day, followed by 200 mg. once daily for 10 to 12 weeks after the CSF has become culture negative. Like CNS toxoplasma infection, cryptococcal CNS infection is associated with a high mortality rate in patients with AIDS.

Herpes simplex virus

Disseminated infection with Herpes simplex virus frequently causes an encephalitis. Typical signs may include lethargy, alterations in level of consciousness, muscle weakness and/or paresis, seizures, disturbances of balance and personality changes. The clinical diagnosis may be confirmed by atraumatic lumbar puncture, which may show the presence of erythrocytes in the CSF and, if necessary, by recovery of the virus (or immunological techniques to demonstrate the virus) from cerebral tissue obtained by brain biopsy (the virus rarely being present in the CSF). The antiviral drug, **acyclovir**, will treat this condition effectively in most patients.

Cytomegalovirus (CMV)

Chorioretinitis, leading to impaired visual acuity in patients with AIDS, is most frequently caused by cytomegalovirus. CMV may also cause encephalitis. CT scans may demonstrate ring-enhancing lesions. The specific medical treatment for CMV conditions is the antiviral drug, **ganciclovir**. **Trisodium phosphonoformate (Foscarnet)** may also be used.

Mycobacteria and *Candida albicans*

Both of these opportunists may cause mass CNS lesions (CT scans showing ring-enhancing lesions). *Mycobacterium tuberculosis* causes tuberculous meningitis or tuberculomas. *Mycobacterium avium-intra-cellulare* may also cause CNS infection. Treatment is with maximum antituberculosis chemotherapy (e.g. **ansamycin, clofazimine, cyclo-**

serine, ethionamide and ethambutol) and, possibly, corticosteroids. Systemic candidiasis, caused by *Candida albicans* may also manifest as meningitis. Fluconazole, amphotericin B (and, sometimes, 5-flucytosine) are used to treat this condition.

Papovavirus (JC virus)

Infection with Papovavirus may cause progressive multifocal leucoencephalopathy (PML) in patients with AIDS. PML has a gradual or insidious onset, the patient frequently presenting with hemiparesis, progressive intellectual impairment, aphasia, dysarthria and hemianopia. CT scans and EEG may be useful in confirming this diagnosis but the definitive diagnostic investigation is identifying the JC virus in brain tissue (obtained by brain biopsy), using immunofluorescence antibody (IFA) staining or electron microscopic agglutination. The course of this disease is relentlessly progressive, the duration from onset of symptoms to death being usually one to four months. Cytosine or adenine arabinoside have been helpful in treatment in a few cases. However, there is currently no effective therapy for most individuals who develop PML.

CNS neoplastic diseases

Approximately five per cent of patients with AIDS develop CNS neoplasms. The most common is B cell lymphomas, usually primary but may be secondary to systemic lymphomas. CNS neoplasms, due to Kaposi's sarcoma, may also occur and cause CNS bleeding.

Space-occupying lesions often present with a history of weakness, lethargy or confusion and focal neurological deficits or seizures.

Diagnostic tests include CT and magnetic resonance imaging scans and examination of CSF fluid. Additionally, brain biopsy may be undertaken. *Toxoplasma gondii* infection may also cause mass lesions in the CNS and this diagnosis should be excluded as it is a potentially treatable CNS infection. Often patients are treated empirically for *T. gondii* infection for a month to see if there is an improvement which may save the patient from requiring a brain biopsy.

Standard anti-cancer drugs (e.g. vincristine, vinblastine and etoposide – VP-16) do not readily cross the blood-brain barrier and treatment consists of total head deep X-ray treatment (DXT) by external beam radiotherapy. Dexamethasone or mannitol and/or diuretics are given to counteract the initial cerebral oedema caused by DXT.

Cerebrovascular disorders

CNS bleeding related to emboli from non-bacterial endocarditis, immune thrombocytopenic purpura (ITP) or cerebral arteritis, is sometimes seen in patients with AIDS.

Onset of symptoms is usually abrupt with headache followed by steadily increasing neurological deficits. Hemiparesis is seen in major bleeds located in the hemispheres. Symptoms of cerebellar or brainstem dysfunction (e.g. conjugate eye deviation or ophthalmoplegia, stertorous breathing, pinpoint pupils and coma) occur when the bleed is located in the posterior fossa. Nausea and vomiting, focal or generalized seizures and loss of consciousness are all common.

The diagnosis is made by CT scans. Lumbar puncture is usually contraindicated as the change in CSF pressure during lumbar puncture may precipitate transtentorial herniation.

Treatment is symptomatic.

Caring for patients with neuropsychiatric syndromes

Actual problems	Origin of problem
Alterations in maintaining self-care requisites	Nervous system dysfunction

Potential problems	
Fever, headache, nausea and vomiting, drowsiness, stiff neck	CNS opportunistic infections and meningeal inflammation

Potential problems	Origin of problem
Alterations in level of consciousness, focal neurological signs, seizures, paresis, personality changes	Cerebrovascular accidents and cerebral dysfunction
Pain, weakness and wasting in arms and legs, flaccidity and atrophy of legs, paraesthesia, facial paralysis	Peripheral neuropathy
Paraesthesia, weakness and spasticity of legs, ataxia, urinary incontinence	Vacuolar myelopathy
Erectile failure, diarrhoea, hypotension	Autonomic neuropathy

Muscular weakness, disorders of
movement   Polyneuropathy

Impairment of reason,
perception,
intuition, memory, language and   Subclinical cognitive
ability to learn   dysfunction

Delirium, dementia, impaired
cognitive function, incontinence   Organic mental disorders

Pressure sores   Incontinence, immobility

Emotional lability   Cerebral dysfunction

Disturbances in gait and   Neuropathy,
sense of balance   cerebellar dysfunction

Airway obstruction   Unconsciousness

Objectives of care
1. Maintain a safe environment in which the patient can recover.
2. Prevent complications from neurological assault.
3. Maintain vital functions; patent airway.
4. Provide support to the patient, family and friends.
5. Assist the patient to regain maximum independence.
6. Assist the patient to meet self-care requisites.

Nursing intervention

Assessment: A functionally-orientated nursing neurological evaluation, as described by Mitchell and Irvin[11] is useful in patient assessment (Table 6.9).

Altered level of consciousness: Information for the nursing assessment will need to be obtained from a variety of sources, including family, friends and neighbours, as the patient will not be able to provide a reliable history. The assessment must take into consideration any medications or non-prescription drugs the patient may be using. A Glasgow coma scale[12, 13] is initiated (see Fig. 6.1) to compare changes in the patient's level of consciousness over a given period of time. This scale assesses three aspects of behavioural response, which indicate the general functioning or dysfunction of the brain. The three aspects of behavioural response assessed are eye-opening, verbal response and motor response.

Table 6.9 Organization of a functionally oriented nursing neurological evaluation

General category	Functional category	Examples of specific function which may be tested
Consciousness	Arousing (reticular activating system)	Arousability, response to verbal and tactile stimuli
Mentation	Thinking (general cortical function plus specific regional functions)	Educational level Content of conversation Orientation Fund of information Insight, judgement, planning
	Feeling (affective)	Mood and affect Perception and reaction to ability, disability
	Language	Content and quantity of speech Ability to name objects Ability to repeat phrases Ability to read, write, copy
	Remembering	Attention span Recent and remote memory
Motor function	Seeing (cranial nerves II, III, IV, VI)	Acuity Visual fields Extraocular movement Pupil size, shape, reactivity Presence or absence of diplopia, nystagmus
	Eating (cranial nerves V, IX, X, XII)	Chewing Swallowing Gag (if swallowing impaired)
	Expressing facially (cranial nerve VII)	Symmetry of smile, frown
	Speaking (cranial nerves VII, IX, X, XII)	Clarity Presence or absence of nasality
	Moving (motor and cerebellar systems)	Muscle tone, mass, strength Presence or absence of involuntary movements Coordination: heel-to-toe walk, observing during dressing Posture, gait, position

General category	Functional category	Examples of specific function which may be tested
Sensory function	Smelling (cranial nerve I)	Ability to detect odours
	Blinking (cranial nerve V)	Corneal reflex
	Hearing (cranial nerve VII)	Acuity, presence or absence of unusual sounds
	Feeling (sensory pathways)	Pain – pinprick Touch, stereognosis Temperature – warm, cold

Eye-opening

Spontaneously – patient opens eyes when nurse approaches bed.
Opening to speech – patient opens eyes in response to his/her name, either at normal speaking voice or increased volume.
Opening to pain – patient opens eyes in response to painful stimuli.
No eye-opening – eyes do not open to speech or painful stimuli.

Best verbal response

Response is recorded to simple, direct questions (light touch or painful stimuli may be used).

Best motor response

Response to commands to raise his/her arm or two fingers is noted. Asking the patient to grasp the nurse's fingers is unreliable as the grasp reflex may still be present.
Ability to localize pain is noted when the patient moves a limb in response to painful stimuli.
Flexion withdrawal to pain occurs when the arm bends at the elbow in response to painful stimuli (e.g. pressure on the patient's fingernail bed).
Abnormal flexion is noted and refers to the arm flexing at the elbow and the turning of the hand so that the palm faces downwards or backwards, making a fist (i.e. pronation).
Abnormal extension to pain occurs when the patient straightens the elbow and moves the arm away from the body (i.e. abduction), often with internal rotation, in response to painful stimuli to the fingernail bed.

Table 6.10   Potential problems relevant to the patient with an altered level of consciousness

Problem	Causative factors	Signs and symptoms
Altered sensation: Visual, auditory, kinaesthetic, gustatory, tactile and olfactory	Abnormal metabolic processes Supratentorial lesions Infratentorial lesions Psychogenic	Disoriented in time or place Disoriented with persons Altered abstraction Altered conceptualization Altered problem-solving abilities Altered behaviour or communication patterns Anxiety Irritability Reports auditory or visual hallucinations.
Alterations in thought processes	Abnormal metabolic processes Supratentorial lesions Infratentorial lesions Psychogenic	Disorientation to time, place, person, circumstances and events Altered perception Lack of concentration Memory deficit Hyper/hypovigilance Impaired ability to make decisions Impaired ability to reason
Airway clearance ineffective	Loss of gag reflex Immobility Impaired perception and awareness	Cough ineffective Rapid respirations Râles and rhonchi present on auscultation of lungs Cyanosis Dyspnoea Secretions in oral pharynx
Impaired physical mobility	Neuromuscular impairment Immobilization Impaired perception or awareness	Altered muscle tone Decreased range of joint movement Impaired coordination Decreased muscle strength

Problem	Causative factors	Signs and symptoms
Potential for injury	Lack of awareness of environmental hazards Potential for complications from invasive therapeutic measures	Bruises and skin abrasions Altered mobility Impaired coordination Disorientation to circumstances and events
Potential impairment of skin integrity	Immobility Altered muscle tone/ spasticity Altered sensation Weight loss Inadequate nutrition Use of restraints, splints, and other devices Urinary incontinence	Redness, oedema, or breaks in skin Immobility Use of restraints, splints or other devices Spasticity Urinary incontinence Decreased sensation
Alterations in nutrition: less than body requirements	Immobility Loss of gag reflex Loss of control of voluntary movement Impaired awareness	Weight loss Decreased daily food/fluid intake Decreased skin thickness Aspiration of food/fluids
Alteration in patterns of urinary elimination: incontinence	Immobility Impaired awareness Sensory motor impairment Neuromuscular impairment	Involuntary voiding
Alteration in bowel elimination: incontinence	Immobility Neuromuscular impairment Impaired awareness Alteration in nutrition	Involuntary passage of stools
Self-care deficit: feeding, bathing/ hygiene, dressing/ grooming, toileting	Impaired perception and awareness Neuromuscular impairment Decreased strength and endurance	Inability to feed, bathe, dress, groom or toilet self Lack of coordination Inability to follow instructions

Pupils.   Pupil size is measured by comparing it to the pupil scale on the chart and pupil reaction is measured in response to light (i.e., a direct beam from an ophthalmoscope or pen light). In health, pupils are of equal size and constrict briskly when stimulated by a direct beam of light.

Limb movement.   Limb movement is assessed by noting the movement of both arms and legs to verbal commands or painful stimuli.
Weakness, either mild or severe, is noted by comparing one limb against the other.
Spastic flexion of the arms is noted if there is a slow, stiff movement of the arm, bending at the elbow and the hand held against the body.
Extension occurs when, in response to painful stimuli, the knee or elbow are straightened.
No response is recorded when there is no movement in response to painful and varied stimuli.

Vital signs.   Vital signs are recorded frequently or continuously monitored. Potential problems associated with unconsciousness have been comprehensively described by Kim *et al.*[14] and are shown in Table 6.10.

Assisting with self-care requisites: Patients with altered levels of consciousness and other manifestations of neurological dysfunction will need assistance with self-care requisites as described in Chapter 9. The need for a safe environment is paramount. Cot sides (bed-rails) are always kept in the upright position for patients with altered levels of consciousness and for patients who are confused. Special attention to the care of the eyes and mouth is vital, as is positioning. Unconscious patients are placed in the lateral or semiprone position and the body properly aligned. Patients must be turned every two hours and pressure area care given. They will require assistance with their need for adequate hydration and nutrition and for faecal and urinary elimination. Frequent reality orientation is essential.

Evaluation: Assistance with all self-care requisites is continuously evaluated and care continued or replanned according to the patient's response and the dynamics of the underlying neuropsychiatric processes.

				Date							
				Time							
GLASGOW COMA SCALE	Eye opening	4. Spontaneously									Eyes closed due to swelling = C
		3. To speech									
		2. To pain									
		1. None									
	Best verbal	5. Oriented									Endotracheal tube or tracheostomy = T
		4. Confused									
		3. Inappropriate									
		2. Incomprehensible									
		1. None									
	Best motor	6. Obeys commands									Usually record best arm response
		5. Localizes to pain									
		4. Flexion/withdrawal to pain									
		3. Abnormal flexion									
		2. Abnormal extension									
		1. None									
	Pupils	Right eye	Size								+ = Reacts − = No reaction C = Eyes closed
			Reaction								
		Left eye	Size								
			Reaction								
LIMB MOVEMENT	Arms	Normal power									Record right (R) and left (L) separately if there is a difference between the two sides
		Mild weakness									
		Severe weakness									
		Spastic flexion									
		Extension									
		No response									
	Legs	Normal power									
		Mild weakness									
		Severe weakness									
		Extension									
		No response									

Pupil scale mm

1 •
2 •
3 ●
4 ●
5 ●
6 ●
7 ●
8 ●

Blood pressure

Systolic = V
Diastolic = ∧
Blue = Lying
Red = Sitting
         Standing

Pulse = •
(Red)

210 200 190 180 170 160 150 140 130 120 110 100 90 80 70 60 50 40

42 41 40 39 38 37 36 35 34 33 32 31 30

°C

Temperature = •
(Blue)

Respirations = •
(Blue)

30 25 20 15 10

30 25 20 15 10

Comments

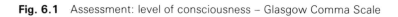

Fig. 6.1 Assessment: level of consciousness – Glasgow Comma Scale

Caring for patients with neuropsychiatric conditions in psychiatric hospitals

Patients may be safely and competently cared for in psychiatric hospitals, when appropriate. This requires aggressive in-service nursing education and the creation of policies and procedures for patients with HIV-related illness which are as thorough as those for district general hospitals.

From time to time it may be necessary to detain patients with neuro-psychiatric syndromes in either district general hospitals or psychiatric hospitals, either to protect them from harm, or more rarely, to protect the community. Patients may be detained in hospital either under the Mental Health Act of 1983 or the Public Health (Control of Diseases) Act of 1984 (inclusive of the statutory regulations made by the Secretary of State on 22 March 1986).

Mental Health Act 1983 (Part II)

The following sections of the Mental Health Act 1983 (Part II) can be used, if required, to detain a patient in hospital.

Section 2:   A patient may be admitted to hospital for assessment, for a period not exceeding 28 days, for either his own health or safety or with a view to the protection of other persons.

Section 4:   A patient may be admitted to hospital for emergency assessment for a period of 72 hours.

Section 5:   Under 5(2), a patient, who is already an in-patient in hospital, may be further detained in hospital for a period of 72 hours. This will allow the consultant in charge to have the patient detained on the ward and will give medical staff an opportunity to decide on further action and, if appropriate, application for detention under other sections of the Mental Health Act.

Further sections of the Act can be used to detain patients for varying periods of time.

Public Health (Control of Diseases) Act 1984

Statutory regulations made by the Secretary of State (22 March 1986) provide for AIDS being a notifiable disease for the purposes of Sections 35, 38, 43 and 44 of the Act. This Act allows for the provisions for compulsory medical examination and for compulsory removal of a patient to hospital, where the interest of the sufferer, his family and the public appear to justify that such action should be taken. Section 38 of the Act allows for the compulsory detention in hospital of a patient already in hospital.

Obviously, the detention of any citizen in hospital against his or her will, is a serious event which, fortunately, is rarely required. However, there are circumstances, when either for the good of the patient or the good of the community, compulsory admission may be appropriate. It may be necessary initially to have the patient evaluated in a district general hospital to rule out treatable neurological syndromes (e.g. opportunistic CNS infections). If the patient is suffering from inter-current psychosis (e.g. depressive or hypomanic phase of an existing manic depressive illness) or if a patient with a chronic psychosis develops AIDS and requires in-patient care, this care is best delivered in a psychiatric hospital.

Clearly, nurses have a profound duty to ensure that the legalities of compulsory admission have been properly enacted and to support the patient, his family and friends during this frightening period.

Long-stay patients in psychiatric hospitals who are infected with HIV are, of course, able to sexually transmit this infection to other individuals. Sexual activity in psychiatric in-patients in long-stay units is probably quite common, perhaps compounded by the effect of chronic psychosis which may diminish judgement and self-control[15]. Considerable vigilance is required from nursing staff to circumvent this risk. The potential risk of violence is always real in individuals who are frightened, confused and have an altered mental state. Excellent guidelines for dealing with violent patients have been produced by the Confederation of Health Service Employees (COHSE) and describe effective measures to both prevent and if necessary, confidently deal with a violent incident[16].

References

1. Wolcott, D.L. (1986). Neuropsychiatric syndromes in AIDS and AIDs-related illnesses, in *What To Do About AIDS: Physicians and Mental Health Professionals Discuss the Issues*, ed. by McKusick, L., Chapter 4, pp 32–44. University of California Press, Berkeley

2. Carne, C.A. (1987). ABC of AIDS: Neurological Manifestations. *British Medical Journal* (30 May), 294:1399–401

3. Ho, D., Rota, T.R., Schooley, R.T., *et al.* (1985). Isolation of HTLV-III from cerebrospinal fluid and neural tissue of patients with neurologic syndromes related to the acquired immunodeficiency syndrome. *New England Journal of Medicine*, 313:1493–97

4. Carne, C.A., *op. cit.*

5. Wolcott, D., Fawzy, F. and Pasnau, R. (1985). Acquired Immune Deficiency Syndrome (AIDS) and consultation-liaison psychiatry. *General Hospital Psychiatry*, 7:280–92

6. Wolcott, D. (1986) *op. cit.*
7. *Ibid.*
8. Asher, D.M. Epstein, L.G. and Goudsmit, J. (1987). Human Immuno-deficiency Virus in the Central Nervous System, in *Current Topics in AIDS, Vol. 1*, ed. by Gottlieb, M.S., John Wiley & Sons Ltd, UK
9. Walton, J. (1985). *Brain's Diseases of the Nervous System*, 9th edition, p 259. Oxford University Press, UK
10. Pohle, H.D. and Eichenlaub, D. (1986). Proposal and preliminary results of a treatment regimen with pyrimethamine, clindamycin and spiramycin (P–C–S) in toxoplasmosis of the central nervous system (CNS), in *Clinical Aspects of AIDS and AIDS-related Complex*, ed. by Staquet, M., Hemmer, R. and Baert, A. Oxford Medical Publications, UK
11. Mitchell, P.H. and Irvin, N. (1977). Neurological examination: nursing assessment for nursing purposes. *Journal of Neurosurgical Nursing*, 9(1):23–28
12. Teasdale, G. (1975). Acute impairment of brain function – Part 1, Assessing conscious level. *Nursing Times*, 71(24):914–17
13. Teasdale, G., Galbraith, S. and Clarke, K. (1975). Acute impairment of brain function – Part 2, Observation record chart. *Nursing Times*, 71(25):972–73
14. Kim, M.J., McFarland, G.K. and McLane, A.M. (Eds) (1984). *Pocket Guide to Nursing Diagnosis*. C.V. Mosby, St Louis
15. Fenton, T.W. (1986). AIDS and psychiatry: practical, social and ethical issues – practical problems in the management of AIDS-related psychiatric disorder. *Journal of the Royal Society of Medicine* (May), 80(5):271–4
16. COHSE (1977). *The Management of Violent or Potentially Violent Patients*. (Report of a special working party offering information, advice and guidance to COHSE members.) Confederation of Health Service Employees, London

Further reading

Price, R.W., and Brew, B. (1990). Management of the Neurologic Complications of HIV-1 Infection and AIDS in *The Medical Management of AIDS*, 2nd ed., Sande, M.A. and Volberding, P.A., editors, W.B. Saunders Co., London

Rosenblum, M.L., Levy, R.M. and Bredesen, D.E. (1988). *AIDS and the Nervous System*, Raven Press, New York, USA

7

Children with HIV Infection

Early in the pandemic, infants and children accounted for only a small number of patients with AIDS. However, as HIV spread into the female population, the number of children with AIDS has increased in countries all over the world. In the United States, an estimated 1500–2000 new HIV infections occur each year in newborns as a result of perinatal transmission, i.e., one child in every 2000 births[1]. By March, 1990, 2,192 cases of paediatric AIDS had been reported to the CDC in the United States and an increase in paediatric AIDS was being reported in all countries in the European Community (EC). For every child with fully expressed AIDS, an additional 2–10 children will be infected, but not yet demonstrating AIDS defining illnesses. As the number of women being infected with HIV is rising each year in all five continents, **one of the largest groups entering the pandemic during the early 1990s will be infants and children**[2].

HIV Transmission to infants and children

The vast majority of infants and children who are infected with HIV have become so as a result of vertical transmission, i.e., from their HIV-infected mothers. Most infants become infected perinatally, either in utero or during delivery **(intrapartum)**. The frequency for successful HIV transmission from an infected mother to her child varies in different parts of the world but on average, the vertical transmission rate is 30–40 per cent[3]. The fetus can become infected in **utero** as early as the 13th week of pregnancy[4].

A smaller (and decreasing) number of children have become infected via contaminated blood products or blood transfusions and rarely, newborn children may become infected in the early postpartum period from infected breast milk[5]. Injecting drug use in very young children has been reported which may expose them to HIV infection. HIV transmission to small children as a result of sexual abuse has also been documented[6].

The misuse of injectable drugs is the primary risk factor for HIV infection among women. More than half of infected women contracted

HIV infection either directly by using blood contaminated injecting equipment, or indirectly through heterosexual contact with infected injecting drug users[7]. The explosion of cocaine (and its derivative, 'crack') use is also associated with increased high-risk sexual behaviour and may be responsible for exposing even more women to HIV infection.

Definition of paediatric AIDS/HIV infection

By definition, paediatric AIDS or HIV infection refers to children under the age of 13 years. Serological diagnosis of paediatric HIV infection is fraught with difficulties. All children born to HIV positive mothers will also be antibody positive for HIV because of the normal maternal transfer of antibodies in untero. Therefore, a standard HIV antibody test for IgG antibodies (e.g. ELISA, HIV immunoassays, etc.) is not a reliable indicator of infection in infants **until after the age of 18 months**. However, during this early period, HIV infection in the infant may be serologically diagnosed by a combination of tests, including virus cultures, antigen detection (usually p24), complete Western Blot analysis and polymerase chain reaction tests (PCR). These tests are described in more detail in Chapter 14. Virus cultures, especially those performed two to three weeks after birth, are capable of identifying up to 80 per cent of children with HIV infection[8]. **It is essential to remember that parents must give true, informed consent prior to their child having a serological test for HIV infection.**

Table 7.1   Principle signs and symptoms in paediatric AIDS

Recurrent and serious bacterial infections
Diarrhoea (persistent or recurrent)*
Oral candidiasis (recurrent, chronic)
Failure to thrive
Lymphoid Interstitial Pneumonitis (LIP)
Serious Opportunitistic Infection, e.g. PCP
Fever*
Parotitis*
Hepatomegaly*
Splenomegaly*
Skin diseases (candidiasis and seborrhea)
Chronic otitis media
Chronic sinusitis
Neurological disease, e.g. acquired microcephaly and/or brain atrophy, progressive symmetrical motor deficits

---

* persisting for more than 2 months

In addition to serological tests, the appearance of clinical symptoms are also important indicators of possible HIV infection in the infant. The main signs and symptoms seen in paediatric AIDS are listed in Table 7.1 and further described in the CDC case definition for AIDS (Table 7.2) and the CDC classification system for HIV infection in children under 13 years of age (Table 7.3), which all paediatric nurses and midwives should be familiar[9].

Table 7.2 CDC case definition for AIDS in children under 13 years of age

For the limited purposes of epidemiologic surveillance, CDC defines a case of paediatric AIDS as a child under 13 years of age who has had:
1. a reliably diagnosed disease at least moderately indicative of underlying cellular immunodeficiency, *and*
2. no known cause of underlying cellular immunodeficiency or any other reduced resistance reported to be associated with that disease.

The diseases accepted as sufficiently indicative of underlying cellular immunodeficiency are:
- Candidiasis of the oesophagus, trachea, bronchi, or lungs
- Cryptococcosis, extrapulmonary
- Cryptosporidiosis with diarrhoea persisting for more than 1 month
- Cytomegalovirus disease of an organ other than liver, spleen or lymph nodes in a child more than 1 month of age
- *Herpes simplex virus* infection causing a mucocutaneous ulcer that persists longer than 1 month; or bronchitis, pneumonitis, or oesophagitis for any duration in a child more than 1 month of age
- Lymphoid interstitial pneumonia and/or pulmonary lymphoid hyperplasia (LIP/PLH complex) affecting a child less than 13 years of age
- *Mycobacterium avium* complex or *M. kansasii* disease, disseminated (at a site other than or in addition to lungs, skin, or cervical or hilar lymph nodes)
- *Pneumocystis carinii* pneumonia
- Progressive multifocal leucoencephalopathy
- Toxoplasmosis of the brain affecting a child more than 1 month of age
- Bacterial infections, multiple or recurrent (any combination of at least two within a two-year period), of the following types affecting a child less than 13 years of age: *
      septicaemia, pneumonia, meningitis, bone or joint infection, or abscess of an internal organ or body cavity (excluding otitis media or superficial skin or mucosal abscesses), caused by *Haemophilus*, *Streptococcus* (including *Pneumococcus*), or other pyogenic bacteria
- Coccidioidomycosis, disseminated (at a site other than or in addition to lungs, or cervical or hilar lymph nodes) *
- HIV encephalopathy *

Table 7.2   *continued*

- Histoplasmosis, disseminated (at a site other than or in addition to lungs or cervical or hilar lymph nodes)*
- Isosporiasis with diarrhoea persisting for more than 1 month*
- Kaposi's sarcoma at any age
- Lymphoma of the brain (primary) at any age*
- Other non-Hodgkin's lymphoma of B cell or unknown immunologic phenotype*

*Indicates a diagnosis of AIDS only if there is also laboratory evidence of HIV infection

Specific conditions that must be excluded in a child are:
1. Primary immunodeficiency diseases – severe, combined immunodeficiency (SCID), DiGeorge syndrome, Wiskott-Aldrich syndrome, ataxia telangiectasia, graft-versus-host disease, neutropenia, neutrophil function abnormality, agammaglobulinaemia, or hypogammaglobulinaemia with raised IgM
2. Secondary immunodeficiency associated with immunosuppressive therapy, lymphoreticular malignancy, or starvation

---

HIV Infection in Adolescents

AIDS and HIV infection also occurs in adolescents (age 13 to 18 years). Young adults presenting with AIDS in their twenties have most likely become infected (either sexually or through injecting substance mususe) as teenagers. Currently, there is an increase in all forms of sexually transmitted diseases in adolescents and in many countries they are a prime target for drug misuse (especially 'crack'). In both the United States and Europe, the majority of adolescents practice high risk sexual behaviour at one time or another[10, 11]. Consequently, a substantial rise in HIV infection in now being seen in teenagers[12]. Adolescents are diagnosed and classified as adults (*see* Chapter 5), however they present more unique legal and ethical problems. Although adolescents can give consent in the United States and in the United Kingdom in all issues involving sexually transmitted diseases, it is far from clear if they can consent to treatment with potentially toxic and in many cases, experimental drugs. It is also not clear if an adolescent can refuse consent to disclose a diagnosis of HIV infection or AIDS to his or her parents.

Table 7.3 Summary of classification of HIV infection in children less than 13 years of age

Class P-0	**Indeterminate infection**

Class P-1   **Asymptomatic infection**
      Subclass A   Normal immune function
      Subclass B   Abnormal immune function
      Subclass C   Immune function not tested

Class P-2   **Symptomatic infection**
      Subclass A   Nonspecific findings
      Subclass B   Progressive neurological disease
      Subclass C   Lymphoid interstitial pneumonitis
      Subclass D   Secondary infectious diseases
         Category D-1   Specified secondary infectious diseases listed in the CDC surveillance definition for AIDS (see pp 91–92)
         Category D-2   Recurrent serious bacterial infections
         Category D-3   Other specified secondary infectious diseases
      Subclass E   Secondary cancers
         Category E-1   Specified secondary cancers listed in the CDC surveillance definition for AIDS (see pp 92)
         Category E-2   Other cancers possibly secondary to HIV infection
      Subclass F   Other diseases possibly due to HIV infection

Classification system

Children fulfilling the definition of HIV infection may be classified into one of two mutually exclusive classes based on the presence or absence of clinical signs and symptoms.

Class Paediatric-1 (P-1) is further subcategorized on the basis of the presence or absence of immunological abnormalities, whereas Class P-2 is subdivided by specific disease patterns. Once a child has signs and symptoms and is therefore classified in P-2, he or she is not reassigned to Class P-1 if signs and symptoms resolve. Perinatally exposed infants and children whose infection status is indeterminate are classified into Class P-0.

Class P-0 (Indeterminate infection)
Includes perinatally exposed infants and children up to 15 months of age who cannot be classified as definitely infected according to the

above definition but who have antibody to HIV, indicating exposure to a mother who is infected.

Class P-1 (Asymptomatic infection)

Includes patients who meet one of the above definitions for HIV infection but who have had no previous signs or symptoms that would have led to classification in Class P-2. These children may be sub-classified on the basis of immunological testing.

Subclass A – Normal immune function includes children with no immune abnormalities associated with HIV infection.

Subclass B – Abnormal immune function includes children with one or more of the commonly observed immune abnormalities associated with HIV infection (see Table 7.4).

Table 7.4   Abnormal immunological findings in infants and children under 15 months who are infected with HIV

increased IgG immunoglobulin levels, anergy (loss of cell-mediated immunity), poor antibody response to antigen challenge, depressed T4 (CD4 +) lymphocyte count, decreased T4(CD4 +)/T8(CD8 +) lymphocyte ratio, absolute lymphopenia

Subclass C – Not tested includes children for whom no or incomplete immunological testing has been done.

Class P-2 (Symptomatic infection)

Includes patients meeting the above definitions for HIV infection and having signs and symptoms of infection. Other causes of these signs and symptoms will have been excluded. Subclasses are defined based on the type of signs and symptoms that are present. Patients may be classified in more than one subclass.

Subclass A – Nonspecific findings includes children with two or more unexplained nonspecific findings persisting for more than two months, include fever, failure-to-thrive or weight loss of more than ten per cent of base-line, enlarged liver (hepatomegaly), enlarged spleen (splenomegaly), generalized lymphadenopathy (lymph nodes measuring at least 0.5 cm present in two or more sites, with bilateral lymph nodes counting as one site), parotitis, and diarrhoea (three or more loose stools per day) that is either persistent or recurrent (defined as two or more episodes of diarrhoea accompanied by dehydration within a two month period).

Subclass B - Progressive neurological disease includes children with one or more of the following progressive findings:

1. loss of developmental milestones or intellectual ability;
2. impaired brain growth (acquired microcephaly and/or brain atrophy demonstrated on CT or MRI scans); or
3. progressive symmetrical motor deficits manifested by two or more of these findings: paresis, abnormal tone, pathologic reflexes, ataxia, or gait disturbance.

Subclass C - Lymphoid interstitial pneumonitis includes children with a histologically confirmed pneumonitis characterized by diffuse interstitial and peribronchiolar infiltration of lymphocytes and plasma cells and without identifiable pathogens, or, in the absence of a histologic diagnosis, a chronic pneumonitis – characterized by bilateral reticulonodular interstitial infiltrates with or without hilar lymphadenopathy – present on chest X-ray for a period of at least two months and unresponsive to appropriate antimicrobial therapy. Other causes of interstitial infiltrates are excluded (e.g. tuberculosis, *Pneumocystis carinii* pneumonia, cytomegalovirus infection, or other viral or parasitic infections).

Subclass D - Secondary infectious diseases includes children with a diagnosis of an infectious disease that occurs as a result of immune deficiency caused by infection with HIV.

Category D-1 includes patients with secondary infectious disease due to one of the specified infectious diseases listed in the CDC surveillance definition for AIDS: *Pneumocystis carinii* pneumonia; chronic cryptosporidiosis; disseminated toxoplasmosis with onset after one month of age; extra-intestinal strongyloidiasis; chronic isosporiasis, candidiasis (oesophageal, bronchial, or pulmonary); extrapulmonary cryptococcosis; disseminated histoplasmosis; noncutaneous, extrapulmonary, or disseminated mycobacterial infection (any species other than *Mycobacterium leprae*); cytomegalovirus infection with onset after one month of age; chronic mucocutaneous or disseminated herpes simplex virus infection with onset after one month of age; extrapulmonary or disseminated coccidioidomycosis; norcardiosis; and progressive multifocal leucoencephalopathy.

Category D-2 includes patients with unexplained, recurrent, serious bacterial infections (two or more within a two year period) including sepsis, meningitis, pneumonia, abscess of an internal organ, and bone/joint infections.

Category D-3 includes patients with other infectious diseases, including oral candidiasis persisting for two months or more, two or more episodes of herpes stomatitis within a year, or multi-dermatomal, or disseminated herpes zoster infection.

Subclass E – Secondary cancers includes children with any cancer described below in categories E-1 and E-2.

Category E-1 includes patients with the diagnosis of one or more kinds of cancer known to be associated with HIV infection as listed in the surveillance definition of AIDS and indicative of a defect in cell-mediated immunity: Kaposi's sarcoma, B cell non-Hodgkin's lymphoma, or primary lymphoma of the brain.

Category E-2 includes patients with the diagnosis of other malignancies possibly associated with HIV infection.

Subclass F – Other diseases includes children with other conditions possibly due to HIV infection not listed in the above subclasses, such as hepatitis, cardiopathy, nephropathy, haematologic disorders (anaemia, thrombocytopenia), and dermatological diseases.

The non-specific term 'AIDS-related complex' (ARC) has been widely used to describe symptomatic HIV-infected children who do not meet the CDC case definition for AIDS. This classification system categorizes these children more specifically under Class P-2. Pulmonary disease accounts for most of the morbidity and mortality associated with HIV infection in children. The most common pulmonary conditions seen are pneumonia caused by *Pneumocystis carinii* (PCP) and lymphoid interstitial pneumonitis (LIP). LIP and PCP are difficult to differentiate. In general, children with PCP are more hypoxic and febrile than children with LIP. The only certain way to diagnose LIP is by lung biopsy. The most common opportunistic infections seen in children infected with HIV are PCP, toxoplasmosis, severe herpes simplex virus infection and disseminated cytomegalovirus infection. Severe and recalcitrant mucocutaneous candidiasis is almost always seen in children with AIDS. Over half of all children with AIDS develop severe and/or recurrent pyogenic bacterial infections, the most common pathogens involved are *Haemophilus influenzae*, *Streptococcus pneumoniae*, *Staphylococcus aureus*, *Salmonella* spp.

Involvement of the central nervous system (CNS) is frequent in children with AIDS and may be the first indication of HIV infection. A progressive loss of developmental milestones or arrest in development being the most common early signs and encephalopathy is also frequently encountered.

Anaemia, thrombocytopenia and other haematological disorders are frequently seen and there may be bleeding from mucosal sites.

Other pathology frequently seen in children with AIDS includes cardiovascular disease (e.g. congestive cardiomyopathy and AIDS arteriopathy), skin diseases (e.g. non-specific intermittent eczematoid eruption and candidal dermatitis), gastrointestinal and liver disease (e.g. malabsorption, enterocolitis, pseudomembranous necrotizing jejunitis). Renal disease (e.g. nephrotic syndrome) may also be seen[13, 14, 15].

Treatment of children with AIDS

Aggressive, supportive treatment can decrease both morbidity and mortality in children with AIDS. The treatment programme developed at the Children's Hospital of New Jersey, as described by Connor

Table 7.5 The goals of the multidisciplinary AIDS programme

1. Treat the disease/symptoms of immune deficiency resulting from HIV infection:
   - aggressive treatment of infections
   - nutritional support (total parenteral nutrition, ongoing nutritional assessment)
   - periodic assessment of growth and development
   - regular neurologic examination and testing for evidence of progressive encephalopathy
   - supportive treatment of chronic lung disease

2. Prevent the disease process and treatment regimen from interfering with the development of the child:
   - provide parents with specific information about the condition and treatment
   - assist the parents to understand and manage the illness and its symptoms
   - assist parents to identify and utilize resources within the health care system and the community
   - assist the child in coping with and understanding the illness at an appropriate age level

3. Prevent the illness and its treatment regimens from disrupting the family unit:
   - assist parents to develop an awareness of their rights within the system
   - act as an advocate for the family with schools and other social agencies
   - educate the professional and lay public

Table 7.6   Therapeutic protocol for paediatric HIV infection

---

Vigorous nutritional support
Hospitalize for parenteral feeding, hyperalimentation, or nasogastric tube
feeding

Antimicrobial therapy for intercurrent infection
Hospitalize for parenteral therapy as needed

Short course steroid for interstitial pneumonia
If patient is hypoxic (PO_2 < 65 mmHg on room air)

IV *gamma-globulin*
Full replacement dose every 3–4 weeks

---

et al.[16], serves as a model to provide maximum supportive care and is
described in Table 7.5 and Table 7.6.

As always, paediatric nursing care requires not only the care of the
child but the care of the entire family who will require support throughout the illness of their child. In most cases, the mother is herself infected
with HIV and pregnancy may have caused a previously asymptomatically
infected woman to develop clinical illness. Her care is discussed in detail
in Chapter 9.

The management of children with HIV infection has previously
concentrated on supportive care, i.e., the medical treatment of
developing opportunistic infections and the relevant nursing care. The
nursing care of children with HIV-related conditions is exactly the same
as for any other seriously ill child. Care is assessed, planned, delivered
and continuously evaluated as per the identified health care deficits of
the infant or child. As for any other child, the parents are involved in all
stages of the process of care, including the setting of short-term,
medium-term and long-term goals.

The advent of specific anti-retroviral therapy for HIV infection and
increasing sophistication in the prophylaxis of common paediatric
AIDS-related opportunistic infections, has increased both the length
and quality of life of many infants and children with HIV-related
conditions. It is recognised that paediatric AIDS progresses more
rapidly than adult AIDS; the median survival time from diagnosis to
death is 14 months[17].

Consequently, the earlier an infant is serologically identified as being
infected with HIV, the earlier an improved quality of medical
monitoring, treatment and prophylaxis can be initiated.

In US, French and Italian studies[18, 19, 20] zidovudine (Retrovir –
AZT) was reported to significantly improve the condition of many

children with symptomatic HIV infection. Improvements were seen in growth, weight and height, neuropsychological function and immunological status. Children with early symptomatic disease tolerated zidovudine well, neutropenia being the main side effect. Although the paediatric dose for zidovudine has not yet been established, a daily dose of 5 mg/kg[21] and twice daily administration may be sufficient[22].

The above studies are currently being extended to establish if zidovudine treatment during pregnancy can prevent **in-utero** (or **intrapartum**) HIV transmission to the fetus. In addition, they are exploring the efficacy of zidovudine treatment within 24 hours of birth to neonates born to HIV-infected mothers in interrupting HIV transmission.

Other anti-retrovial agents are now in various phases of clinical studies[23] and hopefully during the early 1990s, increasingly effective and specific treatment for this disease will evolve. Zidovudine and other anti-retroviral drugs are discussed more fully in Chapter 14.

Immunisation and children infected with HIV

Children infected with HIV are at an increased risk from infectious diseases and should be vaccinated as a matter of priority. They should follow the approved schedule for routine immunisations as given in Table 7.7. Vaccine efficacy may be reduced in children who are infected with HIV and they may additionally need passive immune protection from the use of human normal immunoglobulin (HNIG) or specific immunoglobulins. If a HIV infected child is receiving full-replacement therapy with intravenous gamma-globulin (i.e., HNIG), an immune

Table 7.7 Routine immunisation schedule UK/1990

Vaccine	Age
diptheria, tetanus, pertussis (DTP) and polio (OPV or IPV)	2 months (1st dose) 3 months (2nd dose) 4 months (3rd dose)
measles, mumps, rubella (MMR)	12–18 months
Booster diptheria and polio	4–5 years
rubella	10–14 years (girls only)
Booster tetanus and polio	15–18 years

Table 7.8 General contra-indications to vaccination

immunisation should not proceed in children who:
have had a severe or general reaction to a preceding dose (all vaccines)

are hypersensitive to eggs (influenza vaccine)

have had previous anaphylactic reaction to eggs (MMR, influenza, yellow fever)

are suffering from an acute illness and are febrile (all vaccines)

are suffering from vomiting and diarrhoea (polio)

response to live virus vaccines (e.g. MMR, polio) may be reduced. **Children who are infected with HIV may safely have all of the vaccines listed in Table 7.7** (as can adults), providing that there are no clinical contra-indications to immunisations, as described in Table 7.8.

In the UK, children who are asymptomatically infected with HIV may receive live polio vaccine (OPV) vaccine) but excretion of the vaccine virus in the faeces may continue for longer than in normal individuals. Household contacts should be warned of this and the need for strict personal hygiene, including hand-washing after nappy changes for an HIV-positive infant. Inactivated polio vaccine (IPV) is generally used for children with symptomatic HIV infection, although OPV may be used.

In developing countries where the incidence of poliomyelitis remains high, the lack of evidence of side effects to OPV support the WHO policy for its continued administration to all children.

In the United States, IPV is recommended for children with both symptomatic and known HIV asymptomactic infection, i.e., OPV is not used.

Table 7.9 lists other vaccines which HIV infected children may receive, if necessary.

In the United Kingdom (and the United States), the Bacillus Calmette-Guerin (BCG) vaccine used for primary prevention of tuberculosis is never given to children (or adults) known to be infected with HIV as serious vaccine dissemination has been reported. However, in

Table 7.9 Vaccines safe to use in HIV-infected children

typhoid	hepatitis B
cholera	influenza
meningococcal	pneumococcal
H. influenzae type b conjugate (HbCV)	

developing countries where the risk of tuberculosis is high, BCG vaccination at birth is still recommended by the WHO.

Yellow fever vaccine is also **not given** to children (or adults) known to be infected with HIV.

It is axiomatic that parents must give true, informed consent prior to their child being immunised. Mothers who know that they themselves are infected with HIV or who have children being investigated for HIV infection, are extremely anxious in relation to immunisations for their children. Nurses who care for these children should have a clear understanding of current recommendations[24, 25].

References

1. Centers for Disease Control (1990). Estimates of HIV Prevalence and Projected AIDS Cases: Summary of a Workshop, October 31–November 1, 1989, *MMWR* (February 23), **39**(7):110–119
2. Heymann, D.L., Chin, J. and Mann, J.M. (1990). A Global Overview of AIDS, in *Heterosexual Transmission of AIDS*, (ed.) Alexander, N.J., Gabelnick, H.L. and Spieler, J.M., Wiley-Liss, New York
3. Bradbeer, C. (1990). Human immunodeficiency virus and its relationship to women, editorial review, *International Journal of STD and AIDS* (July) **14**:233–238
4. PHS – National Institute of Child Health and Human Development (1990). *The New Face of AIDS: A Maternal and Pediatric Epidemic* (June) U.S. Department of Health and Human Services
5. WHO (1987). Global Programme on AIDS on Special Programme of Research, Development and Research Training in Human Reproduction: Joint Statement – *Contraceptive Methods and HIV Infection*, SPA/INF/87.9, Geneva
6. Rubinstein, A. and Bernstein, L. (1986). The epidemiology of pediatric acquired immunodeficiency syndrome, *Clinical Immunology and Immunopathology*, **40**:115–21
7. PHS – National Institute of Child Health and Human Development (1990). *op. cit.*
8. Rouzioux, C. (1989). Methods of Early Diagnosis, in *Aspects of Paediatric HIV Management* (International Seminar Series), ed. by McFadzean, W., pp 14–18, Colwood House Medical Publications (UK)
9. Centers for Disease Control (1987). Classification System for Human Immunodeficiency Virus (HIV) Infection in Children Under 13 Years of Age, *MMWR* (April 24), **36**(15):225–32
10. DiClemente, R., Durbin, M., Siegel, D., Krasnovsky, F. and Lazarus, N. (1990). An inverse relation between number of sex partners and condom use frequency among middle adolescents: Cause for concern, *VI International Conference on AIDS – Abstracts*, Th.D.897, San Francisco
11. Nieuwinckel, St., Knops, N., Poppe, E. and Van Hove, E. (1990). Belgian Adolescents and AIDS – A Survey of Risk Behaviour and Prevention, *VI*

International Conference on AIDS - Abstracts, Th.D.776, San Francisco

12. Kilbourne, B.W., Chus, S.Y., Oxtoby, M.J. and Rogers, M.F. (1990). Mortality due to HIV infection in adolescents and young adults, *VI International Conference on AIDS - Abstracts*, Th.C.743, San Francisco

13. Cilleruelo, M.J. (1990). Clinical Disease Spectrum, in *Aspects of Paediatric HIV Management* (International Seminar Series), ed. by McFadzean, W., pp 19-26, Colwood House Medical Publications (UK)

14. Grossman, M. (1990). Special Problems In The Child With AIDS, in *The Medical Management of AIDS*, 2nd ed., Sande, M.A. and Volberding, P.A., editors, W.B., pp 385-397, W.B. Saunders Co., London

15. PHS - National Institute of Child Health and Human Development (1990). *op. cit.*

16. Connor, E.M., Minnefor, A.B. and Oleske, J.M. (1987). Human Immunodeficiency Virus Infection in Infants and Children, in *Current Topics in AIDS (Volume 1)*, (ed.) Gottlieb, M.S., Jeffries, D.J., Mildvan, D., *et al.*, Chapter 9, p 193, John Wiley & Sons, UK

17. PHS - National Institute of Child Health and Human Development (1990). *op. cit.*

18. Griscelli, C. (1990). The French Zidovudine Open Study, in *Aspects of Paediatric HIV Management* (International Seminar Series), ed. by McFadzean, W., pp 33-36, Colwood House Medical Publications (UK)

19. Wilfert, C. (1990). Review of US Clinical Trials, in *Aspects of Paediatric HIV Management* (International Seminar Series), ed. by McFadzean, W., pp 37-41, Colwood House Medical Publications (UK)

20. Giaquinto, C. (1990). Italian Experience and Future Trials, in *Apsects of Paediatric HIV Management* (International Seminar Series), ed. by McFadzean, W., pp 42-45, Colwood House Medical Publications (UK)

21. Griscelli, C. *loc. cit.*

22. Giaquinto, C. *loc. cit.*

23. Johnson, R.P. and Schooley, R.T. (1989). Update on antiretroviral agents other than zidovudine, in *AIDS*, **3**(suppl 1):S145-151, Current Science Ltd., UK

24. Centers for Disease Control (1988). Immunization of Children Infected with Human Immunodeficiency Virus - Supplementary ACIP Statement, *MMWR* (April 1), **37**(12):181-182

25. Department of Health, Welsh Office, Scottish Home and Health Department (1990). *Immunisation against Infectious Diseases* - 1990, HMSO, London

8

A Strategy for Infection Control in Nursing Practice

It is axiomatic that in assessing and planning strategic nursing care for patients with an infectious disease, an extensive understanding of appropriate infection control (IC) procedures is required. Comprehensive guidelines for infection control have been published in both the United Kingdom and the United States and all nurses should be fully conversant with these documents[1,2,3]. The CDC Recommendations for the prevention of transmission of HIV (and other bloodborne pathogens) in health care settings are re-printed in full in Appendix 3 of this book. The information in this Chapter is compatible with this guidance and is in a large part based on guidelines issued by the UK Departments of Health in 1990[4].

The concept of 'Universal Precautions'

With the escalating numbers of individuals presenting for care who are asymptomatically infected with HIV (or other bloodborne viruses, e.g. hepatitis B, hepatitis C, delta hepatitis, etc.), it will never be known with any great certainty who is infected and who is not infected. Even if all in-patients were serologically screened for markers of HIV infection on admission, this procedure could not reliably detect all those who are asymptomatically infected (see Chapter 14). The only certainty that exists is that for the rest of our professional lives, more and more individuals will become infected and an ever increasing number of these individuals will require health care.

Universal Precautions embraces the concept that the blood and certain body fluids of all patients are considered potentially infectious for bloodborne pathogens. Table 8.1 lists the body fluids to which **Universal Precautions** apply. **Blood is the single most important source of potential HIV infection in health care settings.** Table 8.2 lists body fluids/excretions to which **Universal Precautions** *do not* apply in relation to the occupational transmission of HIV in health care settings. However, since some of the fluids and excretions listed in Table 8.2 represent a potential source for nosocomial and community-acquired

Table 8.1   Universal Precautions apply to:

blood
cerebrospinal fluid
peritoneal fluid
pericardial fluid
pleural fluid
synovial fluid
amniotic fluid
semen
vaginal secretions

any other body fluids containing visible blood

saliva in association with dentistry
unfixed tissues and organs

Table 8.2   Universal Precautions do not apply to: (unless containing visible blood)

faeces*
urine *
nasal secretions*
sweat
tears
vomitus*
saliva*

*may contain other potential pathogens

infections with other pathogens, nurses **should not** be handling faeces, urine, nasal secretions, saliva or vomitus *without wearing gloves.*

Risk of HIV infection after exposure

Although the risk of occupational acquisition of HIV in health care settings is extremely low, it does exist and cases have now been documented where health care workers have become infected as a result of occupational exposure[5]. It is sad to note that the very first documented case of a nurse becoming infected with HIV as a consequence of occupational exposure occurred in the United Kingdom[6]. The **major risk** to health care workers is being accidentally inoculated with blood from a patient or client infected with HIV.

Evaluation of the risk of acquiring HIV infection in a health care setting is based upon prospective studies of exposed workers which demonstrate that, on average, the risk of transmission of HIV per episode of percutaneous exposure (e.g. a needlestick or cut with a sharp object) to HIV-infected blood is approximately 0.4 per cent. The risk of HIV transmission per episode of mucous-membrane or skin exposure to HIV-infected blood is less than that following a percutaneous exposure. The risk of HIV transmission following exposure to HIV-infected body fluids or tissues (other than blood) described in Table 8.1 is unknown[7, 8, 9, 10, 11]. Although the risk is low, the risk is real and consequently, the adoption of **Universal Precautions** into current nursing practice is mandatory. This is one of the most fundamental (and radical) changes in nursing practice required by the emergence of HIV. Although **Universal Precautions** are now comprehensively covered in pre-registration nursing programmes, an active strategy for in-service education needs to be developed and implemented to meet the different identified needs of nurses working in general medical-surgical and specialist service areas and in the community.

Virus fragility

There is nothing indestructible about HIV. It can easily be destroyed by a variety of physical and chemical means.

Decontamination methods

Decontamination refers to the methods described in Table 8.3. To assure the effectiveness of any decontamination process, equipment and instruments **must first be thoroughly cleaned.**

Any decontamination method intended to sterilize instruments will of course destroy HIV. Sterilization by **heat** is the most consistently efficient method used and the following procedures are recommended. In hospitals, all sterilizable (non-disposable) instruments are sterilized

Table 8.3 Decontamination methods

Sterilization	Destroys all forms of microbial life, including high numbers of bacterial spores
High-level disinfection	Destroys all forms of microbial life, except high numbers of bacterial spores
Intermediate-level disinfection.	Destroys Mycobacterium tuberculosis, vegetative bacteria, most viruses and fungi but does not kill bacterial spores
Low-level disinfection	Destroys most bacteria, some viruses, some fungi, but not Mycobacterium tuberculosis or bacterial spores

by saturated steam under pressure in an **autoclave** at 2.2 bar, 134 degrees Celsius, maintained for a minimum of three minutes. Alternative autoclave temperatures and hold times are 121 degrees Celsius for 15 minutes or 115 degrees Celsius for 30 minutes. **Hot air sterilizers** can also be used as long as the centre of the load achieves and maintains a temperature of either 180 degrees Celsius for 30 minutes or 160 degrees Celsius for one hour. **Ethylene oxide gas (EOG)** may be used to sterilize delicate instruments. For EOG to be effective, instruments must be both clean and dry as excessive moisture can create residue which can be hazardous. Several methods used in High, intermediate and low level disinfection processes will also easily inactivate HIV. The most useful are:

Boiling: HIV can be inactived by boiling at 100 degrees Celcius for five minutes.

Chemical Disinfectants: Most disinfectants, if used according to the manufactures instructions, are easily able to inactive HIV. The most common chemical disinfectants used which are effective in inactivating HIV are:-

2% alkaline glutaraldehyde is used for non-corrosive disinfection of delicate instruments, e.g. fibreoptic endoscopes. To be effective, the instruments must be thoroughly cleaned prior to disinfection and the gluteraldehyde must be freshly activated. Instruments which will enter sterile body cavities are immersed in glutaraldehyde for a minimum of 3 hours. Other instruments need only be immersed for 30 minutes {unless *M. tuberculosis* is a suspected contaminant, in which case, the instrument is immersed for a minimum of 60 minutes}[12].

Fresh aqueous solutions of sodium hypochlorite (bleach) or **sodium dichloroisocyanurate** are commonly used as general surface disinfectants. **Strong solutions** of sodium hypochlorite (i.e., 10,000 parts per million {ppm} of available chlorine) are used for blood or body fluid spillages. This is equivalent to household bleach diluted 1 part bleach to 10 parts water. Community nurses who use household bleach to make up a sodium hypochlorite solution should be aware that the strength of individual brands of bleach may vary and that hypochlorite may deteriorate with age. **Weak solutions** of sodium hypochlorite (i.e., 1 000 ppm of available chlorine) are used for general disinfection when surfaces are *not* contaminated with visible blood or body fluids. Granular sodium dichloroisocyanurate (e.g. 'Presept') is ideal for blood or body fluid spillages. Both sodium hypochlorite and sodium dichloroisocyanurate are left in contact with the surface being disinfected for two minutes[13].

Other chemical disinfectants which inactivate HIV include hydrogen peroxide, chlorhexidine gluconate and povidone-iodine solutions. Although alcohols can inactivate HIV, they are slow acting and are therefore not recommended[14]. If used, instruments must be thoroughly cleaned and then immersed in either 70% isopropanol alcohol or industrial methylated spirits for a minimum of one hour[15].

Universal Precautions in Nursing Practice

The adoption of **Universal Precautions** in clinical nursing practice requires the implementation of the practice points described in Table 8.4. Specific infection control practice points relevant to the nursing

Table 8.4 Universal Precautions

1. Hands must be washed before and after all patient contact procedures. Nurses who have cuts or abrasions must ensure these are covered with a water-proof dressing.
2. Good quality, non-sterile, disposable latex gloves and plastic aprons are worn when handling blood, body fluids, excretions or secretions from any patient, including patients with HIV-related illness. Gloves are also worn when touching non-intact skin or handling equipment soiled with blood and body fluids. Gloves are changed after contact with each patient
3. Masks and protective eyewear (or face shields) and long-sleeved gowns are worn during procedures which may generate droplets of blood or other body fluids or when there is gross environmental contamination of blood, body fluids, excretions or secretions. Clearly this will be required in midwifery and operating departments
4. Hands must be washed immediately (preferably with a povidone-iodine scrub, e.g. 'Betadine' or a chlorhexidine gluconate solution, e.g. 'Hibiscrub' or 'Hibiclens') if contaminated with blood, body fluids, excretions or secretions from any patient, including patients with known HIV infection
5. Special care is required when handling needles and other sharps. Needles must not be bent or recapped after use and must be discarded immediately into a puncture resistant, waterproof container (e.g. 'Sharps Disposal Bins' – Daniels Health Care Products Ltd)
6. Local policy may still require that all specimens from patients with known HIV infection are sent to the laboratory with a hazard warning on them (e.g. 'Biohazard', 'Risk of Infection'). With the universal implementation of 'Universal Precautions' for all patients, this should no longer be necessary
7. Spillages of blood and other body fluids should be covered with granules of NaDCC (sodium dichloroisocyanurate), such as 'Presept' granules, left for a few minutes and then carefully wiped up with disposable paper towels or scooped up with a scooper

care of all patients, including those known to be infected with HIV (or other blood-borne pathogens) include the following:

Ward accommodation: There is no infection control justification for allocating single room accommodation to patients with HIV infection simply because they are infected with HIV. Quite clearly, with the large number of individuals in the community currently infected with this virus, hospitals will not have single room accommodation for all patients who have AIDS, let alone for all patients who may be sero-positive for anti-HIV. There is no reason why patients with AIDS and HIV-related conditions cannot be nursed on an open ward with complete safety. The nursing assessment of each patient will dictate whether or not a single room is required. Table 8.5 summarizes the indications when a single room is useful. As many patients with AIDS will have nursing care issues outlined there, it is clear that a single room *will* frequently be required. However, there is a difference between a patient admitted with Kaposi's sarcoma for a biopsy (who does not require a single room) and a seriously ill patient admitted with a host of opportunistic infections. Patients not admitted to single rooms can move about freely on the ward and other than for **Universal Precautions**, do not require any restrictions. The major disadvantage of admitting a patient into a single room is the further sense of isolation and rejection felt by most patients with HIV-related conditions. As is usual, all nursing care must be planned with the patient. Careful explanation of IC precautions must be given to the patient. If a patient is admitted to a single room, this does not necessarily mean that the patient is *confined* to that room. For example, patients with diarrhoea may be allowed full ward activities as appropriate.

All patients in single room accommodation must be frequently re-

Table 8.5 Indications for single room accommodation

1. Patients who have an opportunistic infection which normally requires a single room (e.g. pulmonary tuberculosis or salmonellal infection)
2. Patients who are bleeding, likely to bleed (e.g. thrombocytopenia, candidal oesophagitis) or who have open or draining wounds
3. Grossly incontinent patients or those with severe diarrhoea
4. Neurological manifestations of HIV infection (e.g. confusion) which make it difficult for the patient to cooperate and maintain good standards of hygiene
5. Patients with conditions associated with excessive, productive coughing
6. Seriously ill patients who require high dependency nursing care
7. Terminally ill patients
8. Psychological or social reasons

assessed. The plan of care for each shift must allow time for nurses to talk to patients, rather than just entering the room when there is something to do. Efforts must be made to ensure that domestic and catering staff are aware of the IC precautions (*not* the diagnosis!), that meals are delivered and the room cleaned. The final responsibility for the patient's environment is a nursing responsibility.

Protective clothing. When a patient is admitted to a single room, health care workers do *not* need to wear *any* protective clothing when entering the room just to talk to the patient, deliver meals, post, newspapers, etc. When entering a room to deliver direct nursing care such as assisting a patient to bathe, dealing with bed-pans, urinals or specimens, recording routine observations, changing dressings or dealing with incontinence, the *only* protective clothing necessary is a disposable plastic apron and a pair of disposable latex gloves.

Gowns are *not* usually required, unless the patient is grossly incontinent. Additional protective clothing is sometimes indicated, such as when dealing with spillages, assisting with invasive procedures (e.g. bronchoscopy), or managing a patient care situation in which there is likely to be a gross environmental contamination with blood or body fluids (e.g. a patient with haematemesis) or extensive draining wounds. In these circumstances, the following protective clothing is indicated: water repellent gowns, latex gloves, a mask and protective eyewear.

Most patients with HIV infection are also excretors of CMV and a mask and eye protection are appropriate in caring for patients who are coughing excessively, although the ability of patients to excrete significant amounts of CMV by coughing is not known. Some patients with AIDS have pulmonary tuberculosis and, in this condition, a mask is required. It may be more appropriate for *the patient* to wear a mask, for instance, when being transported to another department for investigations or treatment, in which case it is unnecessary for health care workers to do so also.

Appropriate disposable gloves are usually those made out of rubber latex, *not* plastic examination gloves. Research has shown that rubber latex gloves are vastly superior to plastic vinyl gloves and consequently, only latex gloves should be used[16, 17]. There is significant variability in the quality and watertightness of all gloves; they should be changed regularly during long procedures and hands washed thoroughly after glove removal. Suitable face masks are high filtration types used in surgery, not flimsy, tissue thin paper masks. Eye protection devices should not resemble underwater goggles. Simple plastic or normal-looking glasses with plain glass lenses are available. If health care workers already wear glasses, they do not need to wear additional eye protection. In general, if a face mask is required, eye protection should be worn.

Catering staff do not need to wear any protective clothing to deliver meals. Housekeeping and domestic staff need only wear a plastic apron and a pair of disposable gloves when cleaning the room. Physiotherapists should wear gloves, plastic apron, eye protection and a face mask when giving chest physiotherapy. Social workers and other members of the hospital staff need not wear any protective clothing. Medical staff follow the same IC guidelines as those described for nursing personnel.

In general, visitors require no protective clothing, unless they are assisting in patient care activities with nursing personnel, who will advise them appropriately.

In patients who have pulmonary involvement, the nurse in charge will be able to advise other health care workers and visitors when a face mask is required.

As pneumonia caused by *Pneumocystis carinii* is one of the most common opportunistic diseases seen in patients with AIDS, it is worth stressing that this particular condition is not infectious to health care workers and others who have a normal immune response.

Injections and sharps. Probably the *only* time the nurse faces a significant potential risk of infection with HIV is when giving injections, caring for intravenous infusion sites or dealing with blood-contaminated sharp instruments, *especially needles*. Disposable syringes and needles must be used and gloves are worn when giving injections or caring for infusion sites and when handling any contaminated sharp instruments. Needle-locking syringes or one-piece needle-syringe units should be used.

Needles must not be re-inserted into their original sheaths or bent after use. It is generally unnecessary to detach the needle from the syringe after use and needles and syringes should be promptly discarded as one unit, into a rigid, puncture-proof plastic container, which is kept by (or taken to) the patient's bedside. When the 'sharps container' is three quarters full, it is sealed, labelled appropriately (e.g. 'Risk of Infection' or 'BioHazard') and sent for incineration. The one exception is that when either venesectionists or medical staff take blood, they must remove the needle from the syringe before ejecting it into the specimen container to prevent a microscopic aerosol spray. Sharps containers must not be constructed of cardboard and must meet DHSS specifications[18]. The range of sharps disposal bins manufactured by Daniels Health Care Products[19] are currently the best sharps containers on the market in the UK.

Bed pans and urinals. Most patients will be able to use toilet facilities in their room. It is not necessary to pour disinfectants into the toilet after use; routine cleaning by housekeeping or domestic staff (wearing gloves!) is all that is required. If bed pans or urinals are used, they should be emptied as per the usual ward procedure by nursing staff (wearing plastic aprons and gloves). Clearly each patient requires his own individual bed pan and urinal, which may be emptied into the patient's toilet, taking care not to splash the contents, and then rinsed. It is not necessary to soak the bed pan or urinal after use in any disinfectant. They should be stored dry in the patient's room. Bed pans and urinals may also be emptied into a 'bed pan washer,' making sure that the door is securely closed before turning on the machine. Disposable bed pans and urinals that require crushing for disposal (e.g. papier mâché products manufactured by Vernaid) offer added advantages over re-usable bed pans and urinals in convenience, safety and patient satisfaction and, in the long term, are more cost effective. Disposal machines must be in good working order and serviced regularly. Many patients with AIDS will have profuse diarrhoea and if they are not able to use their own toilet, a bedside commode is preferable to using a bed pan in bed.

Linen. If *visibly* contaminated with blood, body fluids, excretions or secretions, from any patient, including patients with known HIV-related conditions, linen is double-bagged. It is first placed in a *red*, plastic bag (preferably an 'alginate-stitched' or polyvinyl alcohol bag), which is then placed into a *red* nylon bag. In the National Health Service (UK), all linen placed in *red* nylon bags is infected linen and no other labelling is required. Hospital laundries have their own procedure for dealing with infected linen, which, since HIV is sensitive to heat and detergents, is usually washed separately in hot, soapy water at a temperature of 71°C for 25 minutes. If the temperature is increased, the duration of the wash may be decreased. A disinfectant, such as hypochlorite, is often added.

Rubbish. Used dressings, paper towels, tubing, and other rubbish visibly contaminated with blood, body fluids, excretions or secretions, from any patient, including patients with known HIV-related conditions is placed in a heavy-duty plastic bag, sealed, and sent for incineration. In the National Health Service (UK), contaminated rubbish placed in *yellow* plastic bags is always incinerated. Additional labelling is not required. When disposing of intravenous tubing, great care must be taken by nursing personnel to ensure that needles and other sharps have first been removed. This may require careful cutting off of *both* sharp ends. Patients who are not in a single room, may dispose of their rubbish (e.g. newspapers,) in the ordinary way, as long as it is not contaminated by blood or other body fluids. In the National Health Service (UK), non-infectious rubbish is disposed of in *black* plastic bags.

Crockery and cutlery. Patients with HIV infection do not generally require disposable crockery and cutlery. In those situations where the patient has a severe mouth infection, pulmonary tuberculosis, or an enteric infection, it is preferable that they use their own normal crockery and cutlery, which can be kept in the patient's room. Often the patient, or the patient's visitors, can assist in washing these few dishes and silver or it can be done by nursing personnel. Rarely are disposable crockery and cutlery needed.

Instruments. Used instruments should be placed in a plastic bag or a special plastic box before being returned to the Central Sterile Supply Department (CSSD) for resterilizing. Instruments which cannot be autoclaved (e.g. endoscopic instruments), should be carefully washed with a detergent to remove all blood and body fluids and then placed in glutaraldehyde 2% for three hours, then rinsed and stored dried. Although HIV can be easily inactivated by most disinfectants, as patients with AIDS frequently have several opportunistic infections, disinfectants which are mycobacteriocidal are used for disinfecting all instruments which cannot be autoclaved. The hospital's specific procedure for using these disinfectants (or the manufacturer's instructions) must be meticulously followed. The advice of the Control of Infection Nurse should be sought if there is any confusion about how these agents should be used.

Contaminated surfaces. Surfaces which may have been contaminated during procedures (e.g. dressing trolleys, tables, and bench surfaces), should be wiped with a *weak* solution of hypochlorite (1000 ppm of available chlorine – e.g. household bleach diluted 1 part bleach to 100 parts of water) or freshly prepared glutaraldehyde 2% (NB hypochlorite is corrosive to metal surfaces and fabrics). Grossly contaminated surfaces should be cleaned with either glutaraldehyde 2% or a *strong* solution of hypochlorite (10 000 ppm – a 1 in 10 dilution of household bleach) which should, where possible, be left in contact with the contaminated surface for 30 minutes, prior to being wiped up with disposable paper towels. An improved method of dealing with spillages of blood or body fluids is to sprinkle granules of NaDCC (dichloroisocyanurate), for example 'Presept' granules over the spillage and after a few minutes, wipe up with disposable paper towels or scoop up with a scooper.

Handwashing. Hands must be washed before and after all patient contact, thus avoiding the introduction of new potential pathogens to an already immunocompromised patient and to prevent transmitting opportunistic microorganisms to other patients. Iodophors (complexes of iodine and solubilizers) such as povidone-iodine ('Betadine', 'Videne') are appropriate as these halogenated soaps have been shown to eradicate HIV[20, 21], and are effective against a wide range of potential pathogens. Chlorhexidine based disinfectants (e.g. 'Hibiscrub', 'Hibiclens') will also readily inactivate HIV.[22] The use of gloves does not eliminate the need for good handwashing techniques.

Table 8.4 summarizes the standard IC precautions that are used with patients who have AIDS or are known to be infected with HIV. **These same IC precautions apply to all patients, regardless of what is known or not known regarding their status for HIV infection!** When a patient is admitted, after a nursing history is taken and the original patient care assessment is completed, the nursing care plan will reflect an adaptation of the above general IC guidelines for each individual patient. All patients with AIDS are not the same. It is not appropriate to have a rigid procedure for AIDS patients, which is implemented without modification each time a patient with this condition is admitted.

Needless to say, patients admitted to hospital for assessment who do not have fully expressed AIDS, but have ARC or are seropositive for anti-HIV, do not require extensive IC precautions. They only require **Universal Precautions**, as described in Table 8.4.

Because of the vast numbers of individuals in the community who are currently infected with this retrovirus and are unaware of it, nurses will often be caring for patients in which the infection is unidentified. Therefore it is essential to adopt sensible IC procedures for *all* patients. Special care must now be taken to avoid contamination with blood and body fluids from *every* patient. Strict attention must be paid to good handwashing techniques, wearing gloves when dealing with *all* blood and body fluids. Diligent care when dealing with needles and other sharps has now become even more obligatory in nursing care. With the advent of AIDS, the days of nurses adopting a casual approach to blood and body fluids from any patient are gone forever. If a nurse or other health care worker has a parenteral (e.g. needlestick or cut) or mucous membrane (e.g. splash to the eye or mouth) exposure to blood or other body fluids, the instructions in Table 8.7 should be followed.

Nurses or other health care workers who have cuts, abrasions or any type of skin lesion, should ensure that these are covered with a waterproof dressing, and that gloves are worn when caring for any patient in whom it is anticipated that exposure to blood or other body fluids may occur.

Table 8.6 Standard IC precautions – AIDS and ARC

Precaution	Procedure	Rationale
1. Single room	Used for patients with .severe diarrhoea, excessive coughing, some opportunistic infections, seriously or terminally ill, bleeding or anticipated bleeding, enteric infections, or for psychological or social reasons	To protect the immunocompromised patient from nosocomial infections, and to protect health care workers and other patients from infection with HIV and associated opportunistic pathogens
2. Plastic aprons and gloves	Used when delivering direct patient care, handling specimens, or domestic cleaning	As above
3. Gowns, masks and eye protection.	Only used in dealing with gross contamination or assisting with invasive procedures, or when the patient is coughing excessively, or at any time in which aerosol contamination is anticipated. Masks without eye protection, either worn by the patient outside the room, or by health care workers inside the room, are required during the early treatment phase for patients with pulmonary tuberculosis	To protect health care workers from infection with HIV or other associated opportunistic pathogens (e.g. *Mycobacterium tuberculosis*, CMV) To protect health care workers from acquisition of *M. tuberculosis* infection
4. Handwashing	Hands are washed prior to, and after all patient care activities	To protect the immunocompromised patient from

Precaution	Procedure	Rationale
	If gloves are worn, hands must still be carefully washed prior to gloving, and after gloves are removed	nosocomial infection and to protect health care workers from acquisition of HIV and associated opportunistic pathogens
	Povidone-iodine 7.5% in a non-ionic detergent base ('Betadine' or 'Videne' surgical scrub) or chlorhexidine gluconate 4% containing isopropyl alcohol 4% detergent ('Hibiscrub' or Hibiclens') is preferred	To prevent transmission of potential pathogens to other patients
5. Needles, injections, and other sharps	Needles are not recapped, bent, or broken after use and are disposed of immediately in a rigid, plastic, puncture-resistant and waterproof 'sharps container'	Meticulous care is required in dealing with sharps to prevent needlestick injuries with possible HIV acquisition by health care workers
	Sharps container is taken to bedside or left in patient's room	Needles are not broken or snapped off in order to avoid a microscopic aerosol of infected material
	Special care is required for disposing of intravenous infusion sets	If sharp ends are not carefully cut off there is a risk that they will puncture side of plastic disposal bags, and injure ancillary staff
	Used instruments are placed in waterproof plastic bag or plastic box and returned to CSSD for autoclaving	To prevent leakage of blood or body fluids while being transported to the CSSD

Table 8.6   *continued*

Precaution	Procedure	Rationale
6. Linen (visibly contaminated with blood or body fluids, excretions or secretions)	Double-bagged. First placed in red plastic alginate bag, which in turn is placed in a red nylon bag, and then closed securely and sent to the laundry Gloves are worn when handling infected linen	To prevent contamination of housekeeping personnel when transporting linen to laundry, and to protect laundry personnel from contamination by infected linen
7. Contaminated material	All infected rubbish, including dressings, drainage tubing and intravenous fluid administration sets (with sharp ends cut off at both ends!) are placed in a heavy-duty yellow plastic bag, securely closed, and sent for incineration	To protect housekeeping and portering personnel from contamination Scrupulous care must be taken to ensure no sharps are placed in rubbish bags
8. Crockery and cutlery	May use ordinary dishes and silverware A patient who has an enteric or mouth infection, or has pulmonary tuberculosis, may keep individual dishes and silver in room	Disposable crockery and cutlery rarely needed To prevent risk of transmitting opportunistic pathogens to other patients
9. Specimens	Gloves must be worn when handling all specimens Specimen container and specimen request form may be labelled with a suitable warning sticker (e.g. 'BioHazard' or 'Risk	To prevent contamination with infected blood and body fluids, affecting everyone who is handling specimens To alert laboratory personnel of special risk

Precaution	Procedure	Rationale
	of Infection') and transported to the laboratory in an impervious plastic bag	To prevent leakage during transport to laboratory
10. Ward privileges	If ambulatory, patient may have full ward privileges (e.g. may go to TV room, hospital shop, etc.)	To prevent isolation
	Patients with diarrhoea should use their·own toilet	To prevent contamination
	Visitors are to be encouraged	

Table 8.7   Procedure for treating parenteral or mucous membrane exposure to blood/body fluids

1. *Parenteral exposure*:
   - injury should be encouraged to bleed by local venous occlusion
   - this is followed by washing the inoculation site for 5 minutes in running water, using povidone-iodine 7.5% in a detergent base ('Betadine' or 'Videne' surgical scrub), or a 4% chlorhexidine gluconate with 4% isopropyl alcohol detergent (e.g. 'Hibiscrub,' 'Hibiclens') or any soap or detergent if the above are not available.
2. *Mucous membrane exposure*:
   - splashes in the mouth: the mouth should be washed out, using running water
   - splashes into the eye: the eye should be well irrigated with either running water or sodium chloride 0.9%
3. The accident should immediately be reported to the senior nurse in charge and an 'Incident Report' should be made out, fully documenting the accident
4. The nurse should be seen in the Occupational Health Department, or by his or her own physician, who will advise on serological screening for anti-HIV

Table 8.7 *continued*

5. *Serological screening for anti-HIV*: A base-line specimen of blood should be taken and either tested for anti-HIV, or stored frozen. Further specimens of blood are tested at 3 and 6 month intervals following exposure.
6. The nurse should be examined and health status documented every six months for one year following the accident. This also provides an opportunity to offer reassurance.

Summary

It is difficult to legislate in policy specific infection control procedures that apply to the variables of clinical nursing practice. **Universal Precautions** require a change in attitude, an acceptance of the concept that whatever IC procedure is appropriate for a patient or client known to be infected with HIV is also appropriate for every patient, in every clinical situation, all the time. Nursing staff have to be involved in the creation and ownership of new IC policies which incorporate **Universal Precautions**. These policies must then be supported by senior nurse managers who are ultimately responsible for ensuring that a procedural basis for a safe working environment is established. The days of having separate IC policies and procedures for patients known to be infected with HIV has long past.

References

1. Centers for Disease Control (1987). Recommendations for Prevention of HIV Transmission in Health Care Settings, *MMWR̀*, (August 21) **36**(2S):3-S-18S
2. Centers for Disease Control (1988). Update: Universal Precautions for Prevention of Transmission of Human Immunodeficiency Virus, Hepatitis B Virus and other Bloodborne Pathogens in Health Care Settings, *MMWR*, (June 24) **37**:377–388
3. UK Health Departments (1990). *Guidance for Clinical Health Care Workers: Protection Against Infection with HIV and Hepatitis Viruses, Recommendations of the Expert Advisory Group on AIDS*, HMSO, London
4. *ibid.*
5. UK Departments of Health (1988). *AIDS: HIV-infected health care workers*, Expert Advisory Group on AIDS, HMSO, London
6. Anonymous (1984). Needlestick transmission of HTLV3 from a patient infected in Africa [editorial], *Lancet* (15 December), **ii**(8416):1376–7

7. Marcus, R. (1988). Cooperative Needlestick Study Goup. Surveillance of health-care workers exposed to blood from patients infected with the human immunodeficiency virus, *New England Journal of Medicine*, **319**:1118–23

8. Henderson, D.K., Fahey, B.J., Saah, A.J., *et al.* (1988). *Longitudinal assessment of risk for occupational/nosocomial transmission of human immunodeficiency virus, type 1 in health care workers* [Abstract] in: Program and abstracts of the twenty-eight interscience Conference on Antimicrobial Agents and Chemotherapy (Los Angeles), Washington, DC: American Society for Microbiology, 221

9. Gerberding, J.L., Littell, C.G., Chambers, H.F., *et al.* (1988). *Risk of occupational HIV transmission in intensively exposed health-care workers: follow-up*, [Abstract] in: Program and abstracts of the twenty-eight interscience Conference on Antimicrobial Agents and Chemotherapy (Los Angeles), Washington, DC: American Society for Microbiology, 169

10. Elmslie, K., Mulligan, L., O'Shaughnessy, M. (1989). *National surveillance program: occupational exposure to human immunodeficiency virus (HIV-1) Infection in Canada*, [Abstracts] V International Conference on AIDS, Montreal, Th.A.P.46, p 148

11. McEvoy, M., Porter, K., Mortimer, P. *et al.* (1987). Prospective study of clinical, laboratory and ancillary staff with accidental exposures to blood or body fluids from patients infected with HIV, *British Medical Journal*, **294**:1595–7

12. UK Departments of Health (1990). *op. cit.* p 40

13. Bloomfield, S.F., Smith-Burchnell, C.A. and Dalgleish, A.G. (1990). Evaluation of hypochlorite-releasing disinfectants against the human immunodeficiency virus (HIV), *Journal of Hospital Infection*, **15**(3):273–278

14. Hanson, P.J., Gor, D., Jeffries, D.J. and Collins, J.V. (1989). Chemical inactivation of HIV on surfaces, *British Medical Journal*, **298**, 862–864

15. UK Departments of Health (1990). *loc cit.*

16. Korniewitcz, D.M., Laughon, B.E., Cyr, W.H., *et al.* (1990). Leakage of virus through used vinyl and latex examination gloves, *Journal of Clinical Microbiology*, **28**(4):787–788

17. Kotilainen, H.R., Brinker, J.P., Avato, J.L. and Gantz, N.M., (1989). Latex and vinyl examination gloves: quality control procedures and implications for health care workers, *Archives of Internal Medicine*, **149**(12):2749–2753

18. Department of Health and Social Security (DHSS) (1982). *Specification for Containers for the Disposal of Used Needles and Sharp Instruments*, Specification No. TSS/S/330.015

19. Daniels Health Care, 130 Western Road, Tring, Herts., HP23 4BU (Telephone: 044 282 6881)

20. Martin, L.D., McDougal, S. and Loskoski, S.L. (1985). Disinfection and inactivation of the human T-lymphotropic virus type III/lymphadeno-pathy-associated virus, Journal of *Infectious Diseases*, **152**:400–403

21. Asanaka, M. and Kurimura, T. (1987). Inactivation of human immuno-

deficiency virus (HIV) by povidone-Iodine, *Yonago Acta Medica*, **30**(2):89–92
22. Montefiori, D.C., Robinson Jr., W.E., Modliszewski, A. and Mitchell, W.M. (1990). Effective inactivation of human immunodeficiency virus with chlorhexidine antiseptics containing detergents and alcohol, *Journal of Hospital Infection*, **15**(3):279–282

Recommended Further Reading

Wilson, J. and Breedon, P. (1990). Universal Precautions – A New Approach to Infection Control, *Nursing Times* (12 September), **86**(37):67–68
Crow, S. (1989). *Asepsis, The Right Touch (Something Old is Now New)*, The Everett Companies, USA

9

The Individualized Care of Patients with AIDS

Patients admitted for investigation or treatment of HIV infection and associated opportunistic disease may be in a rapidly changing clinical situation. Therefore nursing care must be assessed, planned and evaluated on a daily basis. This requires a comprehensive understanding by the nurse of the rationale which underpins strategic nursing care.

Strategic nursing care is that care which is developed and implemented by Registered Nurses, designed to meet the immediate needs of patients, solve identified actual problems and prevent recognized potential problems from being realized. Because of their training and experience, their comprehensive understanding of the nursing issues involved, and their teaching and management skills, Registered Nurses are able to assess and plan the individualized nursing care most appropriate for each patient, leading and supervising the nursing team implementing this care. Care delivered must be evaluated frequently (often on a shift-by-shift basis) and modified according to the patient's response to nursing intervention. The Registered Nurse is ideally placed to act as the patient's advocate and to liaise effectively between the patient and other members of the health care team.

Strategic nursing care embraces the concept of a problem-solving approach to the individualized care of each patient. However, it is more than a nursing process style of care. It includes assessment and planning of nursing care on a hospital-wide basis, taking into consideration all the real and possible issues governing the implementation of care and includes both logistical, educational and managerial aspects, which, if not anticipated, may preclude the delivery of individualized, high quality care. In this chapter we are going to explore planned care for individual patients; further chapters will discuss the issues and back-up nursing support required to deliver this care effectively.

Strategic nursing care: a model for patients with HIV-related disease

Behavioural models of nursing, as conceived by Henderson[1], Roper[2] and Orem[3], are valuable tools by which individualized nursing care of patients with HIV-related disease can be planned and implemented efficiently and effectively. These models describe needs and self-care requisites necessary for normal, healthy living. The use of these models allows for the speedy identification by the nurse of unmet needs and deficits in self-care requisites. A nursing assessment includes the recognition of unmet needs and actual problems. It further identifies potential problems associated with the patient's condition (social, psychological, physical and medical), specific illness, hospitalization and medical treatment. Identifying and documenting needs, self-care requisites, actual problems and potential problems facilitates planning appropriate nursing intervention and allows the effectiveness of this intervention to be evaluated. In discussing the strategic nursing care of patients with HIV-related disease, an eclectic approach to behavioural models of nursing has been used. The overall objective of planned nursing care is to 'assist the individual, sick or well, in the performance of those activities contributing to health or its recovery (or to peaceful death) that he would perform unaided if he had the necessary strength, will or knowledge. And to do this in such a way as to help him gain independence as rapidly as possible'[4].

Needs

In common with all individuals, patients with HIV-related disease have needs which they or others must meet for health to be maintained. Table 9.1, adapted from Henderson's **Components of basic nursing**[5] and Roper's **Activities of Living**[6] lists the needs which may be examined during the nursing assessment. By examining these requisites

Table 9.1　Requisites for health

1. The need for adequate respiration
2. The need for adequate hydration
3. The need for adequate nutrition
4. The need for urinary and faecal elimination
5. The need to control body temperature
6. The need for movement and mobilization
7. The need for a safe environment
8. The need for personal cleansing and dressing
9. The need for expression and communication
10. The need for working and playing
11. The need for adequate rest and sleep
12. The need to maintain psychological equilibrium
13. The need to worship according to own faith
14. The need to express sexuality
15. Needs associated with dying

or needs, problems may be identified. These may be either current problems (actual problems) or problems that may be anticipated due to the patient's need deprivation, medical condition or treatment (potential problems).

1. The need for adequate respiration

Potential problems
Dyspnoea, cough, tachypnoea, cyanosis

Origin of problem
Pneumonia (*Pneumocystis carinii*, CMV other opportunistic pathogens)
Neoplastic involvement from Kaposi's sarcoma or anaemia

Objectives of care
1. To maintain optimal respiratory function.
2. To alleviate cough.
3. To keep patient well oxygenated.

Nursing intervention

Assessment: Vital signs (blood pressure/pulse/respiratory rate/body temperature), arterial blood gases (ABG), colour, respiratory effort, chest sounds, sputum production and mental status should be noted and documented as a base-line assessment.

Position: The patient should be placed in a position which facilitates good respiratory function. Sitting the patient upright, leaning forward and well supported is frequently useful in that it allows the accessory muscles (sternomastoid, pectoralis major, platysma and latissimus dorsi) to assist respiratory effort.

Oxygen: Depending on the patient's clinical condition and arterial blood gases (ABG), the physician may prescribe supplemental oxygen to be administered. In general, the lowest concentration of oxygen needed to overcome hypoxaemia will be ordered. Concentrations of inspired oxygen less than 40% are well tolerated for long periods of time and may be administered by Ventimasks (Vickers Limited Medical Group) or Edinburgh masks (British Oxygen Co. Ltd). Double nasal cannulae may be preferred as they are comfortable and do not interfere with eating, drinking and the wearing of spectacles, although the inspired oxygen concentration provided is unpredictable. An oxygen flow rate of 2 litres per minute will provide approximately a 30% concentration. High concentrations of supplemental oxygen are sometimes required. They can be administered by Polymasks (British Oxygen Co. Ltd) or MC masks (Medical and Industrial Equipment Ltd), both of which deliver approximately a 60% concentration at a flow rate of 4–6 litres per minute. Oxygen administered by these masks requires humidification. Oxygen concentrations of greater than 60%, which have significant toxic effects on the alveolar capillary endothelium and bronchi, should not be used for long periods unless absolutely necessary for the patient's survival. Oxygen therapy should be continuous rather than intermittent, aiming to maintain a constant arterial partial pressure of oxygen (aOPP) between 60 and 80 mmHg.

Patient education: Patients should be taught deep-breathing and coughing exercises. The employment of an incentive spirometer is useful for deep-breathing exercises.

Chest physiotherapy: Extensive chest physiotherapy will be required to assist in establishing and maintaining clear lung fields. Postural drainage is frequently required.

Suction: Patients with severe respiratory embarrassment will require suction. Disposable gloves, plastic apron, high filtration mask and eye protection are necessary when suctioning patients as explosive coughing releases a potentially contaminated aerosol spray.

Medications: Medications are administered as prescribed and potential side-effects should be anticipated. These include:

Medication	*Possible side-effects*
Pentamidine isethionate	Hypoglycaemia (or more rarely, hyperglycaemia)
	Hypotension
NB: test urine twice daily for sugar and acetone. Monitor daily blood glucose estimates (normal: 2.5 – 4.7 mmol/l) (45–85 mg/100 ml)	Abscesses at injection sites – skin rashes Tachycardia Pruritus Thrombocytopenia
Aerosolized pentamidine Trimethoprim- sulfamethoxazole (co-trimoxazole)	Cough and bronchospasm Drug fever Rash Leucopenia

Others: DFMO (difluore-
methylomithine), sulfadoxine
and pyrimethamine and Dapsone

Nausea and vomiting; various
haematological disorders – rash
nephrotoxicity; neurological
disorders

Other medications may be prescribed including **expectorants** (brom-
hexine HCL or mixtures containing either syrup of ipecacuanha,
guaiphenesin or saturated solution of potassium iodide), **cough
suppressants** (mixtures containing either dextromethorphan, codeine
phosphate or pholcodine), and other **antibiotics**.

Reassurance: Patients with respiratory distress require frequent reassurance from the nurse. They are often anxious, tending to panic if they
feel they cannot breathe. The 'nurse call system' should be placed
within easy reach of the patient.

Mouth care: Oxygen is drying to mucous membranes and frequent
mouth care will be required. Patients should rinse their mouth out with
water or a pleasantly flavoured mouthwash solution every hour.

Nasal care: If nasal cannulae are used, it is useful if the anterior nares
are lightly coated with a protective ointment, such as vaseline or
glycerine.

Evaluation: Patients should be reassessed frequently and changes in

- vital signs and body temperature
- colour
- sputum production
- chest sounds
- arterial blood gases

documented. Changes in respiratory status must be reported to the
physician immediately. The patient must also be frequently reassessed
for signs of new chest infections. Frequent measurements of arterial
blood pressure must be made while patients are receiving pentamidine
isethionate.

2.   The need for adequate hydration

Potential problems
Dehydration

Origin of problem
Inadequate intake of oral fluids:
dysphagia secondary to *Candida
albicans* infection or KS lesions,
lethargy, confusion or coma

Fluid loss: diarrhoea, nausea, vomiting, GI suctioning, fever and diaphoresis, hyperpnoea

Electrolyte imbalance   diarrhoea, nausea, vomiting, GI suctioning

Objectives of care
1. To correct dehydration and electrolyte imbalance.
2. To maintain optimal hydration and electrolyte homeostasis.

Nursing intervention

Assessment: The patient should be weighed daily (at the same time each day) and an exact record of fluid intake and output maintained. Skin turgor should be assessed on a daily basis.

Oral fluids: The patient should be encouraged to drink frequent, small amounts of oral fluids as tolerated. For all patients, especially those with fever, a plentiful supply of fresh iced water should be kept on the patient's bedside locker.

Intravenous rehydration: The physician will prescribe a regime of intravenous fluids. These fluids must be infused at the correct flow rate, as ordered by the physician.

Electrolyte replacement: Electrolytes will be added to intravenous infusions according to the physician's prescription. Patients with potassium imbalance may be continuously assessed by using a cardiac monitor.

Mouth care: Dehydrated patients require frequent (two-hourly) mouth care.

Evaluation: Effective rehydration and electrolyte replacement will result in normal skin turgor, blood pressure, heart rate and absence of signs of mental confusion or vertigo (if due to dehydration).
   Plasma electrolyte levels should be carefully monitored and results outside normal parameters reported to the physician immediately.

Normal electrolyte parameters:

Potassium:	3.8– 5.0 mmol/l	(mEq/l)
Sodium:	135–145 mmol/l	(mEq/l)
Chloride:	100–106 mmol/l	(mEq/l)

3. The need for adequate nutrition

Actual problem
Weight loss

Origin of problem
Catabolism associated with
AIDS

Potential problems
Further severe weight loss
and malnutrition

Increased catabolism, fever,
diarrhoea, nausea and vomiting
Profound anorexia
Dysphagia – KS lesions in GI
tract, malabsorption

Objectives of care
1. To keep patient well nourished.
2. To prevent further weight loss.
3. To enhance weight gain.

Nursing intervention

Assessment: Weigh patient and take history of previous dietary patterns, including likes, dislikes and any known food allergies. Note the current dietary habit of the patient as many patients with AIDS will be on special diets, often as 'alternative' forms of treatment (e.g. macrobiotic diets). The dietitian should be informed of the patient's admission and, after interviewing the patient, will be able to advise on a nutritional regime.

Oral nutrition: The patient may tolerate small, frequent meals better than the traditional three meals a day. Every effort should be made to present the patient with food he likes. This can be brought in by visitors if it is not readily available in the hospital. Yogurts and meal substitutes ('Carnation', 'Ensure Plus') are often well tolerated. If allowed by the physician, a small amount of sherry prior to meals may stimulate appetite. Prescribed anti-emetics should be given an hour before meals. Usually the dietitian will advise the nurse on any special diets ordered for the patient. Some patients may wish to follow their own special diet, such as a macrobiotic diet. This may present a conflict as current medical opinion does not feel this diet is useful in a catabolic condition. This can be discussed with the patient but, in the end, his wishes must be respected. He may feel his diet is his only remaining hope.

Enteral tube feeding: Enteral feeding is often employed in AIDS patients who are seriously ill and cannot be maintained on oral nutrition. A naso-gastric tube is passed, usually being left *in situ*. Isotonic, lactose-free formulae are often employed, the solution generally being administered at between 50 and 100 ml an hour, depending on the patient's tolerance of it. Diarrhoea is a severe reaction to enteral feeding but may be controlled by reducing the rate of administration. An alternative regime is to pass a naso-gastric tube, leaving it *in situ* for a morning or an afternoon and only feeding the patient during this time, making up nutritional requirements with either oral or parenteral feeds.

Parenteral nutrition: Solutions of protein, lipids and carbohydrates may be infused intravenously. Trace elements, electrolytes and vitamins may be added. Short-term peripheral parenteral nutrition can be employed, although it is more usual for parenteral nutrition to be administered via a central line. There are risks associated with total parenteral nutrition (TPN). Patients frequently become hyperglycaemic due to the carbohydrate load. Insulin may be added to the solution to control this. All patients on TPN should have four-hourly urinalysis for sugar and ketone bodies as well as daily blood glucose estimates. Great care must be taken of the infusion site and line as they frequently become infected. When TPN is discontinued, it must be done *gradually* and the patient carefully observed for signs of hypoglycaemia.

Medications: **Anti-emetics** are almost universally prescribed for patients with AIDS who have nausea and vomiting. Probably the most frequently used anti-emetic is metoclopramide ('Maxolon'), which can be given either orally or by intramuscular or intravenous injection. Anti-emetic suppositories such as thiethylperazine maleate ('Torecan') may be useful with some patients. **Antidiarrhoeals** may be effective with some patients. However they are notoriously ineffective in many patients with AIDS who have severe diarrhoea. The most common antidiarrhoeals used include diphenoxylate HCL with atropine sulphate ('Lomotil') and loperamide HCL ('Imodium'). Codeine phosphate may also be used. **Supplemental vitamins**: Most patients with AIDS will have vitamin supplements prescribed. Many will be on their own regime of 'mega-dose' vitamin therapy. As fat-soluble vitamins (A,D,E and K) are toxic in high doses, the physician must be aware of any medication the patient has brought in with him and is taking in hospital. This includes vitamin preparations.

Evaluation: If nutritional support is successful, the patient should show a weight gain or, at least, a cessation of weight loss. Unfortunately, weight loss and malnutrition are generally profound, persistent and progressive. The patient must be weighed weekly and recordings of fluid intake and output maintained. Abdominal girth is measured weekly. The patient's abdomen is marked clearly so that all nursing personnel measure the girth consistently. Bowel sounds should be assessed four-hourly when on enteral feeding.

4. The need for urinary and faecal elimination

Potential problems	Origin of problems
Diarrhoea	Opportunistic infections (e.g. cryptosporidiosis, CMV amoebiasis, *Isospora belli*), KS lesions in the GI tract, or of idiopathic origin
Oliguria	Dehydration
Incontinence	Confusion, loss of mobility, terminal illness

Objectives of care
1. To control or minimize effects of diarrhoea and incontinence.
2. To achieve effective implementation of enteric IC precautions, if indicated.
3. To facilitate correction of water imbalance.

Nursing intervention

Assessment: Frequency of bowel movements should be documented and fluid intake and output recorded.

Toilet facilities: Patients with diarrhoea should be nursed in a single room which has private toilet facilities. If the patient is not ambulatory, a bedside commode is preferable to using a bed pan in bed. Bed pans may be carefully emptied (to avoid splashing) in the patient's toilet, or the contents disposed of in the bed pan washer.

Skin care: The skin must be kept clean and dry. It is essential that facilities are made available for the patient to wash his hands after using the toilet. If the patient is incontinent, protective or barrier creams may be useful in preventing excoriation of the skin (e.g. 'Sprilon' spray – Pharmacia GB Ltd, or 'Vitamin A + D Ointment – Emollient' – E. Fougera & Co.).

Hydration: Patients with severe diarrhoea may become quickly dehydrated and the patient must be encouraged to drink adequate amounts of fluids to replace those lost due to diarrhoea. Intravenous rehydration may be necessary in some patients.

Nursing care of the incontinent patient: Urinary incontinence may be managed by leaving an urinal carefully placed between the patient's legs. Alternatively, external catheters, such as the 'Texas' latex penile sheath (Cory Brothers Ltd) or 'Uro-Flow' non-allergenic penile sheaths, with hypo-allergenic, adhesive, distensible foam liners (Downs Surgical Ltd.) may be used. Patients with faecal incontinence should be nursed on clean, dry incontinence pads, which are placed on a linen drawsheet over a plastic sheet. All patients who are incontinent must be checked hourly.

Diet: The dietitian may be consulted in order to assess if a change in the patient's diet may assist in controlling faecal incontinence.

Pressure area care: Patients who are incontinent are at an increased risk of developing pressure sores. Pressure area care, including turning the patient on alternative sides, should be undertaken every two hours. It is useful to reassess the patient daily using the Norton scale[7].

Infection control: Nurses must wear rubber latex disposable gloves (of the correct size!) and plastic aprons when disposing of urine or faeces and when caring for incontinent patients. Contaminated linen is double-bagged in a red plastic bag, which is then placed in a red nylon bag, sealed and sent to the laundry. Careful handwashing, prior to and after caring for patients is exceptionally important with patients who have enteric infections. Wearing gloves does not decrease the need for good handwashing technique. If patients have enteric infections, they should have their own set of crockery and cutlery, which may be kept in the patient's room. This can be washed by the nurse after use. This is preferable to presenting food to a patient with gastrointestinal symptoms on unattractive disposable paper plates and asking him to use plastic knives, spoons and forks.

Evaluation: Effective nursing intervention will prevent dehydration secondary to severe diarrhoea, skin excoriation and pressure area breakdown. It will also help to minimize the psychological effects of severe diarrhoea and/or incontinence.

5. The need to control body temperature

Potential problem   **Origin of problem**
Fever and night sweats   Opportunistic infections

Objectives of care
1. To assist in maintaining normal body temperature (36–37.5°C)
2. To keep the patient comfortable.

Nursing intervention

Assessment: Patients with AIDS and ARC should have vital signs and body temperature recorded four-hourly. The occurrence of night sweats is common in both conditions and should be documented in the nursing notes.

Medication: The physician may prescribe medication to reduce body temperature, such as aspirin or paracetamol BP (acetaminophen USP). These should be administered as ordered.

Comfort: The patient should be kept clean, dry and well hydrated. Prolonged fever increases metabolic processes. The patient should be encouraged to eat a nutritious diet. Glucose drinks, such as 'Lucozade', may be beneficial to some patients, although they may exacerbate diarrhoea in others. Bed clothes and linen should be light, dry and clean. If hyperpyrexia occurs, sponging with tepid water may prove useful. Iced drinks must be available for the patient with fever.

Evaluation: Pyrexia and intermittent fevers should be detected promptly and medication administered as per the physician's orders.

6. The need for movement and mobilization

Potential problems   **Origin of problem**
Muscle atrophy   Restricted mobility
Decubitus ulcers   Weakness and bed rest
Deep vein thrombosis   Catabolism
          Peripheral neuropathy

Objectives of care
1. To prevent the formation of decubitus ulcers and deep vein thrombosis.
2. To minimize muscle wasting.

3. To achieve full mobilization and independence within the limits of
    the patient's abilities.

Nursing intervention

Assessment: The patient's level of independence and ability to
ambulate, along with any signs of muscle wasting, pressure sores or
venous thrombosis will be assessed daily.

Physiotherapy: Patients not confined to bed should be walked frequently and encouraged to be as independent as possible. Patients on
bed rest must have active and passive lower limb exercises and their
position changed every two hours. A pull-rope, attached to the end of
the bed, or a trapeze bar on a bed frame may prove useful with many
patients.

Pressure area care: Patients on bed rest or semi bed rest must have
two-hourly pressure area care. Gentle massage with a lanolin-based
cream ('TLC' cream or Baby Lotion) is soothing to the patient and

Norton's scoring scale					
Patient's name:			Date:		
Physical condition:			**Mental condition:**		
Good	4		Alert	4	
Fair	3		Apathetic	3	
Poor	2	Score: _____	Confused	2	Score: _____
V. bad	1		Stuporous	1	
Activity:			**Mobility:**		
Ambulant	4		Full	4	
Walk/help	3		Sl. limited	3	
Chairbound	2	Score: _____	V. limited	2	Score: _____
Bedfast	1		Immobile	1	
Incontinent:					
Not	4				
Occasionally	3				
Usually/ur.	2	Score: _____			
Doubly	1				
★ ★ ★ Total score:					

Fig. 9.1   Norton's Scoring Scale

Relief of pressure chart				
Date	Time	Position of patient	Relief of pressure achieved by	Nurse's signature
12/11	0800	Lying on back	Turned on left side	W.Jones.
"	1000	Lying on left side	Turned on Right side	E.Karn
"	1200	Lying on right side	Turned on to back	J. baard.
"	1400	Lying on back	Turned on left side	A.Hilton

Fig. 9.2 Relief of pressure chart

allows an opportunity for the nurse to inspect pressure sites. Patients with restricted mobility should be commenced on a Norton scoring scale[8] as illustrated in Fig. 9.1. Patients with a total score of 14 or less are prone to develop pressure sores and patients with a total score below 12 are more likely than not to develop pressure sores.

It is also useful to commence a patient on a 'Relief of pressure chart'[9] as illustrated in Fig. 9.2.

Nursing care must be organized in order to turn the patient every two hours and lifting must be skillful in order to prevent shearing force to the skin. The skin must be kept dry, cool and clean. Dehydration, malnutrition and anaemia are all predisposing factors to the development of pressure sores. When possible, these must be corrected.

Evaluation: Effective nursing care will promote mobilization and independence and result in absence of pressure sores, venous thrombosis and excessive muscle wasting.

7.   The need for a safe environment

Potential problems
Nosocomial infection
Accidents

Origin of problem
Immunodeficiency
Weakness
Confusion
Hospital environment and equipment
CMV retinitis

Objectives of care
1. To prevent nosocomial infection.
2. To maintain a safe environment.

Nursing intervention

Assessment: An assessment of the patient's mental status includes determining his ability to understand and cooperate in his planned care. The patient's physical condition is assessed, including sight, a history of vertigo, seizures, falls and general state of debilitation.

Infection control: Infection control (IC) procedures will be implemented as per the previous chapter on this aspect of nursing care. All patients with immunodeficiency are at increased risk of nosocomial (i.e. hospital-acquired) infection, although patients with AIDS/ARC are more in danger of previously-acquired, latent infection. As patients with AIDS/ARC are at increased risk from new infections, it is essential that when in hospital they are not exposed to the added risk of nosocomial infections.

Safety: The following aspects must be taken into account when care is planned in order to maintain a safe environment:

1. *Oxygen*: When oxygen is in use, cigarette smoking is not allowed and 'Hazard' notices are prominently displayed in the patient's room. If spanners (wrenches) are needed for oxygen tanks, 'non-sparking' wrenches must be used. Heating pads and other electrical appliances are not used.
2. *Equipment*: All equipment must be carefully put away after use so that it does not present a hazard to patients who are ambulatory. It is essential that a clear pathway is maintained between the patient's bed and the toilet.
3. *Miscellaneous*: Floors are kept clean and dry. If patients are confused or sedated, bedside rails are kept in the upright position when the patient is in bed and the bed is kept in the low position. The 'nurse-call system' is always kept within easy reach of the patient.

Evaluation: Effective planned care will reduce potential safety hazards and prevent the patient from acquiring nosocomial infections.

8. The need for personal cleansing and dressing

Potential problems	Origin of problem
Poor oral hygiene	Dehydration
	Infection
	Lethargy
Inadequate body hygiene	Confusion
	Incontinence
	Immobility

Objectives of care
1. To maintain good oral hygiene.
2. To preserve the integrity and cleanliness of the integumentary system.

Nursing intervention

Mouth care: Ambulatory patients should be encouraged to brush their teeth with a soft toothbrush after each meal and taught how to use dental floss or dental tape to keep the teeth clean. Glycerine and lemon swabs may be used. Mouthwash solution is useful for patients who have a dry mouth or halitosis. Candidiasis ('thrush') is a common opportunist infection in patients with AIDS/ARC, requiring treatment with antifungal preparations, such as topical applications of nystatin oral suspension or amphotericin lozenges. In patients with AIDS/ARC, systemic antifungal medication may be needed. **Fluconazole** (Diflucan), either orally or intravenously is commonly used. Candidal oesophagitis may occur as well as disseminated candidiasis in some patients with AIDS.

Body hygiene: The patient should have a daily bath or shower. If confined to bed, a daily bed-bath is required. Patients who are ambulatory should be encouraged to dress in clean outdoor clothes for part of the day. Patients who have fever and/or night sweats may need assistance in washing after an episode of sweating, requiring careful drying and a change of night clothes and bed linen. Talcum powder after washing is often soothing.

Pressure area care: Two-hourly pressure area care is required for patients confined to bed, as described previously.

Infection control: Patients who have skin lesions and cannot use the shower, should have an antibacterial agent, such as Triclosan 2%

('Ster-Zac' bath concentrate – Hough Hoseason & Co. Ltd), in their bath to prevent secondary infection. Personal clothing which becomes contaminated can safely be disinfected by washing in a washing machine with ordinary detergents, on the hot cycle. Patients should have their own toothbrush and razor. These should not be shared with anyone else. An electric razor may be useful, especially if the patient has a bleeding disorder.

Evaluation: The patient remains clean and dry and the integument intact. Candidiasis is controlled.

9.   The need for expression and communication

Potential problems	Origin of problem
Impaired cognition	Neurological consequences of
Disorientation	infection with HIV or CNS
	opportunistic disease
Isolation	Fear of AIDS by family, friends,
	health care workers
	Excessive IC precautions

Objectives of care
1.   To minimize the effects of neurological dysfunction.
2.   To prevent the deleterious effects of social isolation.

Nursing intervention

Assessment: Establish the status of the patient's orientation to time, place and events. Document visitors the patient wishes to see (and any he does not wish to see).

Visitors: Caring for the patient's visitors is often a delicate task, especially if they do not know the patient's diagnosis or sexual orientation. No information on any aspect of the patient's condition may be given to any visitors without the patient's express consent. With the patient's permission, visitors should be encouraged. The special friend(s) or lover of a homosexual patient often assumes the role of the patient's next of kin, which must be respected. As always, all visitors to the hospital must be treated with respect and consistent courtesy. An officious or abrupt manner displayed by health care workers to visitors can do immeasurable damage to their willingness to visit the patient and is demoralizing to the patient. It is also an unpardonable professional transgression. If possible, visitors should be allowed throughout the day. Some patients with AIDS will have been abandoned by both friends and family. With the patient's permission, it is possible to contact voluntary support groups (e.g. the Terrence Higgins Trust) who can arrange for members from their organization to visit the patient. The hospital's voluntary services may also be able to provide this service.

Communication aids: The patient should have easy access to a telephone, stamps and stationery. If in a single room, it may be possible for the patient to have a television set. The patient should have a bedside radio (with earphones), newspapers and magazines. The 'nurse-call system' must always be within easy reach of the patient. There should be a clock and a calendar in the patient's room.

Time for talking/listening/touching: Nursing care plans must take into account the fact that patients need to talk to their nurses. Listening, holding a patient's hand and just quietly being with the patient is a necessary aspect of nursing art.

Infection control: Appropriate IC precautions, as described previously, are necessary for patients who are immunocompromised or infectious. However, excessive IC precautions represent another barrier between the patient and other human beings and must be avoided. When appropriate, the patient should be encouraged to enjoy full ward privileges and to mix with other patients.

Reality orientation: Patients who are confused must be gently reminded of their environment, day and date and reassured that they are safe. They must not be spoken to as if they were children. It is generally useful if first names are used when speaking to the patient unless he has objected to this. There is nothing wrong in nurses using their own first names when talking to patients. Patients often relate better to health care workers when allowed to use their first names rather than using 'Nurse Adams' or 'Miss Williamson'.

Evaluation: A plan of care which is designed to allow patients both space and time to communicate with their families, friends and health care workers will reduce the sense of loneliness, rejection and isolation felt by many patients with AIDS.

10.   The need for working and playing

Potential problems
Economic hardship

Origin of problem
Loss of employment

Mental deterioration   Boredom, CNS involvement,
                                        loneliness

Objectives of care
1. To provide access to appropriate financial resources.
2. To minimize effects of boredom and loneliness.

Nursing intervention

Assessment: Effects of absence from usual employment are assessed
and the nursing history documents the patient's neurological status and
the presence of any sensory deficits or physical disablement. The
history should include information relating to the patient's past leisure
time activities, hobbies and interests. It is important to assess if the
patient expects visits from family and significant others (lover, friends)
or if he has been abandoned.

Financial problems: It is probable that all patients with long term illness, including AIDS, will eventually need to claim various State
benefits to which they are entitled. As the Social Security system is con-
fusing and complex, the patient should be interviewed by a social
worker as soon as possible. Table 9.2 indicates some of the benefits to
which patients may be entitled.

In the UK, individuals with AIDS can obtain information on entitle-
ment from the Department of Health by telephoning the operator and
asking for 'DHSS Freephone' or telephoning the Department of Health
in London on 0 800 666 555. The prompt issue of medical and sick-
ness certificates, while the patient is in hospital, is important and should
not be left until the patient asks for them. The social worker may also be
able to assist patients who have been dismissed by their employers as a
result of illness.

Table 9.2   Benefits (UK)

Sickness Benefit	Severe Disablement
Family Credit	Allowance
Housing Benefit	
Social Fund Loans	Unemployment Benefit
Statutory Sick Pay	
(SSP)	
Attendance Allowance	Social Fund Payments
Mobility Allowance	
Invalidity Benefit	
Income Support	

Leisure time activities: It is important that patients have access to television viewing and a radio. The library services of the hospital should be introduced and arrangements made for the patient to purchase newspapers and magazines. An occupational therapy assessment may be indicated for some patients. Special interests and hobbies should be encouraged.

Visitors: Visiting times must be flexible and visitors encouraged. If the patient has no visitors, with his permission, the Volunteer Services or a voluntary organization may be able to arrange visitors for the patient. The largest voluntary organization in the United Kingdom for patients with AIDS is the Terrence Higgins Trust and they can be contacted by telephone on (London) 071 831 0330 or 071 242 1010. It is also important for the patient to have visits from health care workers, especially if they are being nursed in single rooms. Time must be made available to visit and talk to the patient rather than entering the room to 'do' something.

Evaluation: The patient receives all necessary assistance to deal with claiming benefit entitlements, planning leisure-time activities and arranging for visitors.

11. The need for adequate rest and sleep

Potential problem   **Origin of problem**
Insomnia   Pain, discomfort or anxiety

Objective of care
1. To ensure that the patient has uninterrupted periods of sleep.

Nursing intervention

Assessment: The patient's usual sleeping environment (e.g. own or shared bed) and habits are ascertained. This includes noting the time the patient usually goes to bed, periods of wakefulness during the night and usual time of rising. Any current complaints of pain or signs of anxiety are noted.

Comfort: Noise is a frequent cause of complaint from all patients in hospital. Every effort must be made to eliminate unnecessary noise, especially during the night. This specifically includes loud talking or laughter at the nurse's station. Drinks containing caffeine (tea, coffee, colas) should be avoided after the evening meal and a hot milk drink

('Horlicks') may be useful in helping to settle the patient. If the physician allows, an alcoholic drink may be beneficial. The patient should be assisted to void before retiring and the bed linen should be straightened. Pressure area care and a back rub are also useful in helping the patient relax before retiring. With seriously ill patients, requiring intensive nursing during the night, care should be planned so that all required care is given at one time, allowing the patient two-hour periods of uninterrupted sleep. Most patients in hospital benefit from an afternoon 'rest period' shortly after lunch. Visitors should be asked not to visit during this time.

Medication: Analgesics or night sedation may be prescribed by the medical staff. Night sedation is ineffective if pain is present. Often appropriate analgesia is sufficient to allow the patient to fall asleep. The benzodiazepine group of drugs are the most useful type of hypnotics used and include nitrazepam and flurazepam. Chloral hydrate capsules, methyprylone and chlormethiazole edisylate are sometimes useful if benzodiazepines prove ineffective. Barbiturates should be avoided. Anxiety may have to be treated with anxiolytic medication such as diazepam, chlordiazepoxide or lorazepam. Early morning wakening may be a sign of clinical depression, which requires specific treatment with antidepressant medications, such as amitriptyline Hcl, doxepin Hcl or trimipramine maleate.

Evaluation: With well-planned nursing care, patients should obtain adequate rest and sleep while in hospital.

12.   The need to maintain psychological equilibrium

Actual problem	**Origin of problem**
Anxiety	Stress associated with progressive, terminal illness, fear of loss of confidentiality

Potential problems	
Ineffective coping	Loss of control
Social isolation	Withdrawal of social supports Isolation in hospital
Loss of self-esteem	Guilt, altered body image, stigma of AIDS, perception of self as contagious to others

Depression   Helplessness, grief associated
                                    with loss of
                                    – personal relationships
                                    – self-esteem
                                    – physical potency
                                    – control
                                    – sexuality
                                    – effective role in life

Objectives of care
1. To allow patient to ventilate feelings and emotions.
2. To alleviate predisposing factors to psychological dysfunction.
3. To offer support.
4. To facilitate referrals to appropriate support personnel/agencies.

Nursing intervention

Assessment: During the first few days of admission, the level of anxiety present can be ascertained. Loss of adequate coping mechanisms and signs or symptoms of clinical depression must be noted. The patient's general affect may change from day to day (or from shift to shift). This must be assessed and documented in order to plan effective nursing intervention.

Anxiety: Anxiety is neither inappropriate nor uncommon in a life-threatening illness such as AIDS. Manifestations of anxiety occur on several levels, ranging from mild tension to sympathetic nervous system overflow and panic. Most patients will require assistance in handling excessive anxiety.

Level 1 (Mild): The patient is alert, enquiring, relatively relaxed and defense mechanisms are working well. In this level, patients are receptive to information.

Level 2 (Moderate): Increased alertness and heightened emotional state. The patient is more receptive to sensory information than factual information and is able to learn relaxation techniques. In this level, patients are able to solve most problems on their own.

Level 3 (Severe): Sympathetic nervous system overflow is present with typical fight-or-flight responses. With severe anxiety, patients are no longer able to solve problems on their own, needing the advocate skills of the nurse. Physical signs and symptoms of anxiety are often present such as tachycardia, restlessness, irritability and a feeling of 'butterflies in the stomach'. The patient is frightened.

Level 4 (Panic):   The patient is overwhelmed by fear – unable to concentrate, having more pronounced physical signs of sympathetic overactivity, such as insomnia, tachycardia, profuse perspiration (especially on the palms and forehead), frequency of micturition and defaecation, rapid breathing and vertigo.

Patients do not progress from level 1 through to level 4, but fluctuate from one level to another. Stressful events occurring during illness may precipitate more severe levels of anxiety. Stressors in AIDS include:

- progressive debilitation
- sensational media interest
- rejection: family, lover, friends, employer
- infection control precautions ('isolation')
- discrimination
- termination of treatment
- required rapid changes in lifestyle
- progressive changes in body image
- threatened (or actual) loss of confidentiality
- growing awareness of prognosis

Intervention designed to alleviate excessive anxiety includes discussing with patients their fears, rationally highlighting their identifiable strengths to cope with stressors, and encouraging socialization and leisure-time activities. Most hospitals have clinical psychologists on their staff who can offer more skilled assistance to the patient in alleviating anxiety and teaching relaxation techniques. Severe anxiety or panic generally requires anxiolytic medication, such as benzodiazepines (discussed previously). These drugs are more useful for short-term management of acute anxiety rather than long-term use.

Depression: Clinical depression is common in AIDS, and its early recognition allows prompt treatment. Patients may despair, complain of sleep disturbances (early morning wakening, difficulty in falling asleep), lose the ability to concentrate, show a loss of interest, energy and further anorexia. Ideas of self-reproach are associated with feelings of despair, hopelessness and guilt. Delusions (false, fixed beliefs) of being punished for being homosexual are common. Loss of sexual interest and impotence is frequent. Suicidal feelings may be articulated, suicide being a significant risk. Mental retardation, as seen in depression, in patients with AIDS often acts as a brake on suicidal acts but it cannot be relied upon. In general, antidepressant medication is required for all but the mildest incidents of depression.

Although there are various types of antidepressants, the **tricyclic** group of antidepressants are the safest and most commonly prescribed.

These include amitriptyline, trimipramine, clomipramine and imipramine. **Tetracyclic antidepressants** are also used, e.g. mianserin hydrocloride (Norval, Bolvidon), maprotiline (Ludiomil) and have less cardiovascular and anti-cholinergic side effects. Another group of antidepressants, known as **monoamine oxidase inhibitors (MAOI)** such as phenelzine, mebanazine and tranylcypromine, are less often prescribed. If a patient is prescribed antidepressant medication, it is imperative that the nurse is aware to which group the drug belongs. MAOIs require specific dietary restrictions as foods rich in tyramine (cheese, Bovril, Oxo, Marmite, chianti and some types of beer) may interact with these drugs and provoke a hypertensive crisis with the risk of subarachnoid haemorrhage. MAOI's also interact with pethidine (meperidine Hcl USP), opiates, phenothiazines and alcohol. In the two to three weeks before antidepressants become effective, the risk of suicide remains real. Antidepressants are generally very effective. Some antidepressants tend to be sedating while others tend to be stimulating. Treatment may have to continue for several months if a relapse is to be prevented.

Patient support groups: A useful way to help patients deal with the various psychological dysfunctions which may occur in AIDS, is to form support groups for those with this diagnosis. These groups are best led by a clinical psychologist who specializes in this condition or by a psychiatric nurse specialist, who has had special training in leading these groups. Following discharge, support groups can be attended on an out-patient basis.

Individual counselling and psychotherapy: In all stages of HIV infection, from seroconversion to fully expressed AIDS and eventual death, individual counselling and psychotherapy will be needed. Although all physicians caring for patients with AIDS will have good counselling and basic psychotherapy skills, the advice and assistance of clinical psychologists will be needed.

Family and significant others: It is not only the patient who requires psychological and emotional support. Family, husbands and wives, lovers and friends all display various levels of anxiety. Enormous demands are commonly made upon nursing staff and the highest degree of skill and sensitivity is required.

Central nervous system disease: HIV can directly cause CNS damage, patients exhibiting signs of a slowly progressive dementia. Gross cognitive changes may occur. The patient will become confused and disoriented. Motor (lower limb weakness) and sensory (blindness) changes may occur. Opportunistic diseases (toxoplasmosis, encephalitis secondary to various opportunistic pathogens, etc.) may also occur, causing a variety of signs and symptoms, all affecting the patient's ability to maintain psychological equilibrium. Some of these diseases are treatable; many are not.

Evaluation: Psychological dysfunction should be recognized early and nursing intervention and medical treatment implemented to alleviate and contain the mental distress which the patient is suffering. Patients will be able to learn to use effective relaxation techniques. Nursing personnel will liaise closely with other care givers.

13.   The need to worship according to faith

Potential problem   **Origin of problem**
Religious deprivation   Isolation, guilt

Objective of care
To facilitate access between patient and chaplain or religious adviser.

Nursing intervention

Assessment: The patient's religious faith and any special religious needs should be ascertained. The patient should be asked if he would like the hospital chaplain to visit him.

Facilitating worship: Chaplains and other religious advisers must, at the patient's wish, have complete access. Often patients can be taken to the hospital chapel for religious services. It is essential that patients have the opportunity of attending confession and of receiving the holy sacraments. The Sacrament of the Anointing of the Sick (i.e. Extreme Unction or Last Rites) is extremely important and this event should be entered in the patient's nursing notes. The sacrament of Holy Communion is important to members of the Church of England and the Roman Catholic Church. At the patient's request, chaplains can make available religious literature and a Bible. The opportunity to participate in religious worship is a tremendous comfort to many patients with AIDS. Patients should not be visited by religious advisers whom they have not requested to see. Many patients, of course, are followers of other, non-Christian faiths and access to their religious advisers is equally important.

Evaluation: The patient will have opportunities to worship and be comforted by his religious beliefs.

14. The need to express sexuality

Actual problem	**Origin of problem**
Need to modify sexual behaviour	Infectious nature of HIV infection

Potential problems	
Loss of libido	Progressive illness
Development of unsafe sexual behaviour patterns	Guilt Internalized homophobia
Grief associated with loss of sexuality	Changing body image, loss of sexual partner

Objectives of care
1. To help patients adjust to changing sexual status.
2. To provide patients with information on safer sex.

Nursing intervention

Assessment: Ascertain patient's attitude towards sexual expression and current problems. Determine patient's knowledge of safer sex techniques.

Patient education: Many patients have immense feelings of guilt over past sexual behaviour, which may have predisposed them to infection with HIV. Christ and Wiener[10] have described five behaviour patterns some patients adopt in response to this guilt:

1. celibacy;
2. denial or rejection of facts leading to continued high levels of sexual activity;
3. celibacy with close friends while engaging in multiple anonymous sexual contacts;
4. increased use of drugs and alcohol;
5. development of small groups of sexual contacts.

Some patients with AIDS have described feelings of internalized homophobia, i.e. an internalization of society's prejudicial attitudes towards homosexuals. This may lead to a belief that homosexuality caused their disease or anger and blame directed at their sexual partner(s).

Reality orientation may reinforce factual information regarding AIDS and its transmission. Some patients need reminding that AIDS is caused by a virus, not by homosexuality, and that, although homosexuals were especially vulnerable to attack by the virus in the first years of the epidemic, *all* sexually active individuals outside of monogamous relationships are at risk. *AIDS is a human disease, not a homosexual disease.* As the vast majority of individuals infected with HIV were infected several years ago before the various 'high risk' sexual activities were identified, no one individual or groups of individuals are to blame for its current pandemic status.

In the current state of knowledge, 'high risk' sexual behaviour is well established. All persons have a responsibility to modify their sexual behaviour accordingly. This includes patients with AIDS, ARC and

Table 9.3 Safer sex guidelines

---

1. **High Risk Sexual Activity**

   Unprotected anal or vaginal sexual intercourse, either active (insertive) or passive (receptive).

   Oral-anal ('rimming') sexual contact. Although it is uncertain if HIV could be transmitted via this activity, new evidence (see Chapter 4) suggests it may be involved in the transmission of a 'Kaposi's sarcoma agent.' It certainly is involved in the transmission of enteric infections and the active partner is most at risk.

   Sharing sex toys (e.g. dildos) and traumatic sexual activity, e.g. manual-anal ('fisting') and sado-masochistic sexual activities (if blood is drawn).

2. **Medium/Low Risk Sexual Activity**

   Protected anal or vaginal sexual intercourse. 'Protected' refers to the male, insertive party wearing a good quality, intact, rubber laxtex condom, preferably one pre-lubricated with nonoxynol-9.

   Performing oral sex on a man who ejaculates into your mouth may be medium or high risk sexual activity.

3. **Low Risk Sexual Activity**

   Performing oral sex on a woman

   Performing oral sex on a man, avoiding ejaculation into the mouth

4. **No Risk Sexual Activity**

   Mutual masturbation

   Erotic touching, caressing and massage

   Kissing and non-genital licking

N.B. Clearly if neither partner is infected with HIV, all of the above activities would be safe from a HIV transmission point of view those who know they are seropositive for anti-HIV. It also includes all sexually active individuals outside of monogamous relationships. Table 9.3 lists current advice for 'safer sex'.

Leaflets explicitly describing safer sex practices are available from both the Health Education Authority (Mabledon Place, London WC1, Telephone 071 383 3833) and the Terrence Higgins Trust (52–54 Gray's Inn Road, London WC1X 8JU, Telephone 071 831 0330). In the United States, this information is available from many organizations including: the San Francisco AIDS Foundation, 333 Valencia St, San Francisco, California 94103, telephone (415) 864 5855 and GMHC, 129 West 20th St., New York, New York 12231, Telephone (212) 807 6664. These may be ordered and stocked on wards or units where patients with AIDS may be admitted and used in patient education programmes. It may be useful to give some patients the telephone number of groups which offer 'safer sex' advice. In the UK, the Terrence Higgins Trust runs an AIDS 'Help-Line' every day on (London) 071 242 1010. In the United States, the Gay Men's Health Crisis (GMHC) have an AIDS 'Hot-Line' on (New York) 212-807 6655. This allows individuals an opportunity independently to obtain information and advice from a source they trust and reinforces patient education efforts in hospital.

If patients are given the right information, most will make the necessary changes in their lifestyle to respond responsibly to the presence of this threat in the community. Some patients with AIDS may have significant psychological dysfunction preventing them from reacting appropriately to health education efforts. In these cases, the nurse should discuss with the attending physician the advantages of a referral to a clinical psychologist who is more skilled in assisting patients adjust to the dynamics of AIDS.

Evaluation: Adequate support and educative efforts will enable the patient to adjust to his changing sexuality and modify future sexual behaviour to protect himself and others.

15.   Needs associated with dying

Actual problems	Origin of problem
Fear, anxiety and loneliness	Impending death, manner of death, loss of power and control

Potential problems	
Physical problems associated with dying from AIDS	Pathophysiology of HIV disease

Inability to adjust to　　　　　Fear
impending death

Objectives of care
1. To alleviate or control physical problems associated with dying from AIDS.
2. To support and reassure the patient through the various psychological stages associated with death.

Nursing intervention

Assessment: Physical problems associated with AIDS affect the dying patient and include:

- pain
- dyspnoea
- nausea/vomiting
- immobility
- open lesions/wounds
- fever

- incontinence
- cough
- pressure sores
- dysphagia
- confusion
- dehydration

In assessing the dying patient, the presence of the above should be noted and care planned accordingly, as discussed previously in this chapter. It is important to ascertain the extent of the patient's knowledge about his own impending death. It is rare that a patient, seriously ill with AIDS, is unaware that he is dying. If his assessment indicates that he is, this fact should be made known to his physician, who has the primary responsibility of discussing the patient's prognosis with him. If (or when) his level of anxiety permits, practical aspects of the patient's death may be gently discussed with him. This may include referral to a legal adviser for patients who have not made a will. It is extremely important that the nursing notes indicate who is to be informed when the patient dies. This information should come from the patient. It would be tragic simply to inform the family, when the most significant relationship may be the patient's lover.

Wills: Patients should be encouraged to make a final and legal will. Patients requiring assistance with this should be directed to the administrative department of the hospital or to the social worker. Under *no* circumstances should nurses help draw up wills or witness them.

Psychological stages of dying: Although it is true that no two individuals react in the same way to impending death, there seem to be commonalities in their reactions. Dr Elisabeth Kubler-Ross has

Table 9.4 The five 'Stages of Dying'

1. **Denial**. 'No, not me.' This is a typical reaction when a patient learns that he or she is terminally ill. Denial is important and necessary. It helps cushion the impact of the patient's awareness that death is inevitable

2. **Rage and anger**. 'Why me?' The patient resents the fact that others will remain healthy and alive while he or she must die. God is a special target for anger since He is regarded as imposing, arbitrarily, the death sentence. To those who are shocked at her claim that such anger is not only permissible but inevitable, Dr Ross replies succinctly, 'God can take it'

3. **Bargaining**. 'Yes me, but . . .' Patients accept the fact of death but strike bargains for more time. Mostly they bargain with God – 'even among people who never talked with God before.' Sometimes they bargain with the physician. They promise to be good or to do something in exchange for another week or month or year of life. Notes Dr Ross: 'What they promise is totally irrelevant, because they don't keep their promises anyway'

4. **Depression**. 'Yes me.' First, the person mourns past losses, things not done, wrongs committed. Then he or she enters a state of 'preparatory grief', getting ready for the arrival of death. The patient grows quiet, does not want visitors. 'When a dying patient doesn't want to see you any more,' says Dr Ross, 'this is a sign he has finished his unfinished business with you and it is a blessing. He can now let go peacefully'

5. **Acceptance**. 'My time is very close now and it's all right.' Dr Ross describes this final stage as 'not a happy stage, but neither is it unhappy. It's devoid of feelings but it's not resignation, it's really a victory'

elegantly described these[13] and Table 9.4 outlines this process.

In reality, patients go back and forth, from one stage to another, not necessarily in consecutive order. However, this model provides a good guide for the nurse in trying to understand the different phases of coming to terms with a terminal illness. In Stage 4, nurses can be helpful in reminding patients of the achievements of their lives, the impact that all human beings have by living a life however short. If the patient has not been abandoned, loved ones have time to express their love and respect, reassuring the patient that he will be remembered.

Last offices: Usual last offices are carried out. The patient is washed and the room tidied. Loved ones are allowed to see the body before further procedures are carried out. The nurse must be accessible during this time as often their grief is close to unbearable. After the body has been viewed, it is placed in a shroud and then gently placed in a heavy duty plastic body bag. Nurses must wear disposable gloves and a plastic apron when carrying out last offices. Once the body has been placed in the body bag, no further IC precautions are required.

Summary

The individualized care of patients with AIDS and HIV-related illnesses requires skill, competence and confidence. These are based on a factual understanding of the pathophysiology of HIV-infection and a comprehensive knowledge of modern models of nursing care, designed to offer all clients, regardless of race, age, creed, sex, sexual orientation or disease, the highest quality of compassionate, nonjudgemental nursing care. Anything less is disreputable to the profession and discreditable to the nurse.

References

1. Henderson, V. (1964). The nature of nursing. *American Journal of Nursing*, 64(8):62–8
2. Roper, N., Logan, W.W. and Tierney, A.J. (1980). *The Elements of Nursing*. Churchill–Livingstone, London
3. Orem, D.E. (1980). *Nursing: Concepts of Practice*, 2nd edition. McGraw–Hill Book Co. New York
4. Henderson, V. (1964). *Basic Principles of Nursing Care*. International Council of Nurses, Geneva
5. *Ibid.*
6. Roper (1980) *op. cit.* p 17–22
7. Norton, D., McLaren, R. Exton–Smith, A. (1975). *An Investigation of Geriatric Nursing Problems in Hospital*. Churchill Livingstone, Edinburgh
8. *Ibid.*
9. Roper (1980). *op. cit.* p 184–5
10. Christ, G.H. and Wiener, L.S. (1985). Psychosocial issues in AIDS, in AIDS: Etiology, Diagnosis, Treatment and Prevention, ed. by DeVita, V.T. Jr., Hellman, S. and Rosenberg, S.A. p 283. J.P. Lippincott Co., New York.
11. Conant, M., Hardy, D., Sernatinger, J., Spicer, D. and Levy, J.A. (1986). Condoms prevent transmission of AIDS-associated retrovirus. *Journal of the American Medical Association* (April 4), 255(13):1706
12. Hicks, D.R., Martin, L.S., Getchell, J.P., *et al.* (1985). Inactivation of HTLV-III/LAV-infected cultures of normal human lymphocytes by Nonoxynol-9 *in vitro*. *Lancet* (December 21/28), ii:1422–3 and Letter – Corrections: Voeller, B. (1986) Nonoxynol-9 and HTLV-III. *Lancet* (May 17), i:1153
13. Kubler-Ross, E. (1969). *On death and dying*. Macmillan, New York

Recommended Reading

Flaskerud, J.H., (ed.) (1989). *AIDS/HIV Infection: A Reference Guide for Nursing Professionals*, W.B. Saunders Co., London

Sims, R. & Moss, V.A. (1991). *Terminal Care for People with AIDS*, Edward Arnold, London

10

Infection Control in Special Departments

Patients with HIV-related illness frequently will be cared for and treated in most departments of the hospital and in the community.

The care of patients in the operating department

With the increasing prevalence of asymptomatic HIV infection in the community, it must be accepted that there will be patients presenting for surgery who are infected with HIV and this will be unknown to operating department personnel (as it will usually be unknown to the patient). Operating theatre nursing practice must be modified to take this important fact into account. The implementation of '**Universal Precautions**' for *all patients, all the time*, regardless of what is or is not known regarding their serological status for HIV infection, will protect both staff and patients while they are in the operating department. The minimum precautions which are now required include the following.

1. Operating department nurses must routinely use appropriate barrier precautions to prevent skin and mucous membrane contact with blood and other body fluids from *all* patients.
2. Plastic aprons should be worn under surgical gowns or gowns used should be made of material that provide an effective barrier against fluid contamination with blood or other body fluids, excretions or secretions.
3. Protective eyewear or face shields should be worn for procedures that commonly result in the generation of droplets, splashing of blood or other body fluids, or the generation of bone chips, regardless of whether or not it is known that the patient is infected with HIV.
4. If a glove is torn or a needlestick or other injury occurs, the gloves should be removed and a new glove used as promptly as patient safety permits. The needle or instrument involved in the incident should also be removed from the sterile field. Needlestick injuries and mucous membrane exposures to blood or other body fluids are dealt with as described in Chapter 8 (Table 8.7).

5. Nursing managers of operating departments must ensure that staff employed to clean contaminated instruments (from *all* cases) consistently wear protective clothing, i.e. intact, heavy-duty rubber gloves, plastic aprons and gowns, and masks and eye protection (or face shield). Eye protection (or face shield) is especially important as the brushing and scrubbing of dirty instruments may cause an aerosol contamination of potentially infected blood and other body fluids.

As previously stated, more often than not, patients infected with HIV will be presented for surgery and their serological status for HIV infection will be unknown. The following IC practice points therefore apply to all patients, all the time.

1. Patients known to be infected with HIV do not need to be placed at the end of the list. There should be adequate time to clean the operating room after each patient.
2. In the anaesthetic room, it is good practice to remove all non-essential equipment from the anaesthetic machine and ventilators, if used, are fitted with a detachable autoclavable circuit and filters.
3. Careful planning is required to ensure that all equipment needed **Universal Precautions** is available. This includes adequate supplies of:
   - appropriate disinfectant (e.g. freshly prepared glutaraldehyde 2%)
   - plastic aprons (which need to be worn under gowns)
   - eye protection devices
   - labels for specimens ('Risk of Infection' or 'BioHazard' labels); if still required by hospital policy
   - red plastic and red nylon linen bags
   - heavy-duty, yellow plastic bags
   - disinfectants for spillages, for example NaDCC granules ('Presept' granules)
   - clear, heavy-duty plastic bags for transport of contaminated ventilators.
4. Non-essential personnel should not be admitted to the operating room during surgery.
5. Circulating nurses in the operating room must wear full protective clothing. This includes gloves (non-sterile), plastic apron, gown, and eye protection.
6. If available, disposable linen should be used for the operating table and trolley. The operating table should be covered with a waterproof sheet, which in turn is covered by a disposable sheet.
7. The patient should be recovered in the recovery unit.

8. All used instruments are carefully cleaned with hot, soapy water, as usual, prior to autoclaving. Personnel responsible for cleaning instruments must wear plastic aprons, gowns, gloves (preferably intact, heavy-duty rubber gloves) and either a mask and eye protection or a face shield.

9. Any spillages of blood or other body fluids should be dealt with as previously described.

10. Non-autoclavable instruments are first carefully cleaned and then soaked in a solution of freshly prepared glutaraldehyde 2% for three hours. It is no longer being recommended that they are first decontaminated by immersing in glutaraldehyde prior to cleaning; the emphasis is now on ensuring that personnel cleaning instruments wear appropriate protective clothing. Regardless of the disinfectant used, the manufacturer's instruction should be precisely followed. If there is any confusion on the proper use of any disinfectant, the senior nurse for infection control should be consulted.

11. Disposable suction jars should be used. These are sealed after use (without first emptying) and discarded into heavy-duty, yellow plastic disposal bags. If non-disposable suction jars are used, 100 ml of sodium hypochlorite 1% (or a NaDCC solution) is poured into the jar prior to use. After use, the contents are emptied carefully, rinsed and autoclaved.

12. Closed circuits from anaesthetic machines or ventilators should be removed and sent to the Central Sterile Supplies Department (CSSD) for decontamination.

13. Ventilators with detachable circuits should be used, for example Penlon Ventilator and Bains Circuit. Only disposable anaesthetic equipment (e.g. airway pieces, masks, corrugated tubing) should be used. It these are not available, only sterilizable equipment must be used.

14. After surgery, the operating room and all equipment must be thoroughly cleaned with hot, soapy water.

15. It is not necessary to allocate a special operating room for patients with HIV infection.

16. Adequate safeguards to protect all patients against unauthorized disclosures must be adopted. Discretion and patient confidentiality must be maintained at all times. This precludes listing the patient's serological status for HIV infection on operating lists which are on general circulation throughout the hospital. It is unnecessary to list any patient's diagnosis or surgical procedure on the operating lists except for the list which remains in the operating theatre.

The care of patients in the out-patients department

Patients with HIV-related illnesses may of course use the reception and waiting room facilities used by all other patients. They do *not* require segregation from patients without HIV-related disease. Venesectionists must wear a plastic apron and a pair of disposable latex gloves when obtaining blood specimens. Endoscopic procedures (sigmoidoscopies, bronchoscopies, etc.) and biopsies do not need to be scheduled for the end of the clinic list. Usual IC precautions are taken when assisting with invasive procedures as described previously. This includes wearing an effective, high-filtration mask, eye protection, a gown over a plastic apron and disposable latex gloves. Suction bottles should contain 30 ml of either glutaraldehyde 2% or a strong solution of hypochlorite.

The care of the patient in the GUM clinic

Many individuals infected with HIV will be initially seen in GUM (Genito-urinary medicine) clinics, which have considerable expertise in dealing with these patients. Because of the epidemic proportions of this infection, sensible IC precautions must be used when dealing with *all* patients seen regardless of their known serological status. This means wearing a plastic apron and a pair of disposable, latex gloves when taking blood from *any* patient in the clinic as well as the adoption of IC precautions appropriate for dealing with sharps, specimens, equipment and all invasive procedures. GUM clinics should be well stocked with explicit health education literature. This can be obtained from the Terrence Higgins Trust in the UK and from either the San Francisco AIDS Foundation or the Gay Men's Health Crisis in the USA. Health advisers play an essential role in supporting these patients. They must have the necessary training and knowledge base in order to do so. There should be a close liaison between the GUM clinic and the Department of Psychology as many individuals require extraordinary counselling and support.

The care of the patient in the maternity service

Antenatal screening
It should be routine for all women attending antenatal clinics to be given information on HIV transmission and offered serological screening on demand. Information on the nature and specific implications of *all* tests performed in pregnancy should be given to the woman concerned and this equally applies to serological testing for the presence of HIV. It is axiomatic that the informed consent of the client must be obtained prior to serological testing.

Counselling

The basic counselling of pregnant women must devolve upon the medical and midwifery staff involved and appropriate staff education on a continuing basis is essential. This should include knowledge of the need and means of obtaining further expert guidance. Additional counselling must be offered to pregnant women for whom a positive serological test for HIV infection is obtained. Some women who have a history of 'high risk' behaviour and have a negative anti-HIV test may also benefit from additional counselling. Such counselling must include advice on safe sexual practice during pregnancy and thereafter.

Termination of pregnancy

Based on the serious consequences of intra-uterine transmission, it is considered that HIV seropositive status is adequate grounds to comply with the requirements of the Abortion Amendment Act 1989/90. Upon confirmation of a positive serological test for HIV infection, the woman must be counselled and given the right to opt for a termination of pregnancy.

With the increasing prevalence of women with asymptomatic HIV infection in the community, modifications in midwifery practice must incorporate **Universal Infection Control** Precautions for *all clients, all the time*, regardless of what is or is not known about their serological status for HIV infection or previous history of 'at risk' behaviour. In assessing and planning for antenatal care, labour and delivery and the postpartum care of all women, the following points should be considered.

Antenatal care

1. *Antenatal diagnostic tests.* Midwives must wear disposable gloves and a plastic apron when taking and handling blood samples from all clients. Extreme care must be taken with needles and other sharp instruments. Needles are never recapped and are disposed of as a single unit (i.e. without detaching the needle from the syringe) into an approved sharps container. The same care is required for all invasive diagnostic procedures (e.g. amniocentesis) involving body fluids.
2. It is not necessary to segregate women known to be infected in the antenatal period unless haemorrhage has occurred, in which case it would seem prudent to implement pre-delivery (intrapartum) care in a single room. However, haemorrhage *in any client* requires **Universal Infection Control Precautions**.
3. Clients should be encouraged to remove their own sanitary towels prior to any procedure or examination. Sanitary towels are

disposed of into a heavy-duty yellow plastic bag (which, when full, is sealed and sent for incineration).

Labour and delivery

1. **Universal Infection Control Precautions** are implemented with *all* clients, all the time. This requires midwifery staff to wear disposable gloves (e.g. surgical rubber latex gloves), effective, high-filtration surgical masks, long sleeve gowns (worn over a plastic apron) and eye protection if there is the possibility of splashing or the generation of an aerosol of blood or body fluids. Protective footwear (boots or plastic overshoes) should always be worn by those directly involved with the delivery, especially for operative procedures when the client is in the lithotomy position. All protective clothing and footwear must be changed before midwifery staff move to other areas within the maternity department.

2. Any cuts or grazes on the hands or arms of midwifery staff must be covered by a closed, unperforated waterproof plaster (tape).

3. If the client is known to be infected with HIV, fetal blood samples, intra-uterine catheters and fetal scalp electrodes should be avoided in order to reduce the risk of transmitting HIV infection to the child.

4. Impermeable forearm protection will be required for intra-uterine manipulation (e.g. manual removal of the placenta).

5. The practice of bleeding the umbilical cord directly into a laboratory tube is out-dated and must be abandoned. The use of a disposable funnel to reduce contamination is the recommended alternative. If a needle and syringe are used, extreme care must be taken to avoid needlestick injury.

6. After examination, the placenta should be placed in a heavy-duty yellow plastic bag, which is sealed and sent for incineration. Hospital policy may require that, any specimens (e.g. cord blood) and the specimen request form from a client known to be infected with HIV is labelled with a hazard warning (e.g. 'BioHazard' or 'Risk of Infection'). However, care must be taken with *all* specimens from *all* clients.

7. Any spillage of blood or other body fluids is carefully covered with NaDCC (dichloroisocyanurate) granules (e.g. 'Presept'), left for five to ten minutes and then carefully wiped up with disposable towels which are then discarded into a heavy-duty yellow plastic bag. Alternatively, the spillage may be saturated with a liquid disinfectant, for example 1% sodium hypochlorite (10 000 ppm

available chlorine) or glutaraldehyde 2%, left for 5–10 minutes and then carefully wiped up as described above. The use of liquid disinfectants for spillages is not as clinically effective as using NaDCC granules as liquid disinfectants require more time in contact with the spillage and their application tends to splash and extend the spillage.

8. Contaminated bench surfaces may be wiped over with NaDCC solution ('Presept') or 0.1% sodium hypochlorite (1000 ppm available chlorine).

Post-natal care

1. After delivery, the health care professional who receives the infant from the midwife should wear a plastic apron under a gown and latex gloves and should continue to wear gloves until the infant is bathed and blood is removed from the skin.
2. After delivery, the mother is returned to the postnatal unit and **Universal Infection Control Precautions** are continued.
3. It is not necessary to have special toilet facilities for use by mothers known to be infected with HIV, however this may be desirable for aesthetic purposes. As all puerperal women have lochial discharge and many have fresh perineal wounds, routine toilet practice in postnatal wards should include the mother wiping the toilet seat with a suitable size disinfectant-impregnated wipe before and after use. The responsibility for wiping the lavatory seat should always be upon the mother about to use it, rather than the preceding user and this feature of postnatal hygiene should be introduced into antenatal education.
4. Showers are preferable to immersion baths. If baths are used, they must be adequately cleaned between use. Triclosan 2% ('Ster-Zac Bath Conc.') may be added to the bath water.
5. If the mother is known to be infected with HIV, she should not breast feed her child as HIV may be transmitted to an uninfected infant via breast milk.

Neonatal care

1. Mouth-operated mucus extractors and mouth-operated devices for the aspiration of blood for fetal scalp sampling are obsolete and must not be used. Instead, for mucus extraction, aspiration should be by means of a syringe, preferably a bulb syringe fitted with a de Lee trap, or by mechanical suction apparatus attached to an 8 or 10 FG suction catheter, using pressure normally not exceeding minus 100 mmHg (minus 136 cm water)[1].

2. After standard management of the cord, the infant should be washed with soap and water (without any antimicrobial agent) in the delivery room to remove all traces of maternal blood and amniotic fluid. Midwifery staff wear protective clothing during this procedure and care is taken to prevent the infant from becoming chilled. Care is also taken to prevent contamination of the cut cord by maternal blood or secretions during cleaning.

3. Disposable napkins should be used and disposed of in heavy-duty yellow plastic bags.

4. Disposable gloves and a plastic apron are worn when taking any blood samples from the baby (including heel pricks) and in routine cord care. Swabs soaked in 0.5% chlorhexidine gluconate in 70% isopropyl alcohol (Hibistat/Hibisol) may be used on the cord stump.

5. The infant should be cared for in the same room as the mother and gloves are worn when dealing with nappy changes or vomit.

6. Scales for weighing all infants should be cleaned between use with 0.5% Chlorhexidine gluconate in 70% isopropyl alcohol (Hibistat/Hibisol) or 0.1% sodium hypochlorite and then wiped with a detergent. Stethoscopes should be cleaned using 0.1% sodium hypochlorite and then wiped with a detergent. After discharge, glass thermometers should be cleaned and then soaked in a solution of 0.5% chlorhexidine and 70% alcohol for 30 minutes.

Caring for patients in the accident and emergency department

The serological status of patients admitted to the accident and emergency department will be unknown to the nursing staff responsible for their care. As large numbers of individuals in the community can be expected to have been infected with HIV, IC precautions designed for HIV infected patients must be adopted for *all* patients requiring examination and treatment. In general, this includes wearing plastic aprons and disposable gloves when exposure to blood and body fluids is anticipated with *any* patient. Obviously 'mouth-to-mouth' resuscitation is never appropriate in a hospital emergency department and resuscitation equipment (airways, endotracheal tubes) should either be disposable or sterilizable, preferably by autoclaving. In emergency situations where gross exposure to blood or body fluids is likely (e.g. serious trauma, haematemesis), gowns (with a plastic apron worn underneath), gloves, masks and eye protection should be worn.

Caring for patients in the intensive care unit

The risk of exposure to blood or body fluids is increased in intensive care units and all of the IC precautions previously described must be implemented. Maximum use should be made of disposable equipment. Non-disposable equipment must be sterilizable. It can no longer be assumed that any blood or body fluid from any patient is 'safe', i.e. HIV-free, and reasonable IC precautions should be incorporated into the planned care of *all* patients. Vascular access sites on *all* patients should be covered with a waterproof dressing. Diligent care must be taken with *all* sharps. The manufacturer's instructions should be followed in sterilizing ventilation equipment.

Summary

There are two important issues to consider in assessing, planning and implementing the nursing care of patients with HIV-related illnesses in the various special departments of the hospital.

1. All departments can safely and competently care for any patient suffering from an infectious disease (including HIV infection) by adopting the general IC precautions outlined previously. In some departments, they will require modification and elaboration, depending on the level of anticipated risk of exposure to blood and body fluids.
2. It should now be clear that it is no longer appropriate to assume that blood or body fluids from any patient are risk-free. Regardless of the known HIV serological status of the patient, routine IC precautions must be implemented for *all* patients, aimed at preventing nursing personnel coming into direct contact with blood or body fluids.

References

1. MacDonald, M.G. (1990). Infection Control Considerations for Management of the Newborn in the Delivery Room, *Pediatric AIDS and HIV Infection: Fetus to Adolescent* 1(1):16–17

11

Discharge Planning and Community Care

Almost all patients with AIDS will require community nursing services at some point in their illness. Successful community nursing care is in part dependent upon good discharge planning procedures when clients are in hospital.

Discharge planning

Effective discharge planning requires strategic planning by hospitals and health authorities. Several issues must be addressed:

Discharge policy

Just as there is often an admissions policy, there must be a discharge policy. Table 11.1 can serve as a model for this policy[1].

On admission, the nursing assessment must include the relevant social history of the patient. This would include an assessment of the **requisites for health** described in Chapter 9 which can then be reassessed and documented upon discharge. A standard format can be used to detail the social history aspects of the nursing assessment if it is carefully designed so that it can be individualized for each patient. The Social History Form in Appendix 4 outlines some of the essential information that a social history must elicit. This form can also serve as a permanent record of the patient's discharge plans.

Procedures for safe discharge should be established and should include guidance for hospital nursing personnel, community nursing personnel and for local authority staff. Following is a suggested model for effecting the safe discharge of patients with AIDS and HIV-related conditions.

Hospital nursing personnel

1. A Social History Form can be initiated in the out-patient's department or the accident and emergency department by the nurse effecting the admission. It remains the responsibility of the nurse

admitting the patient to the ward to complete the form as far as possible during the initial nursing assessment.

2. The nurse in charge of the ward is responsible for ensuring that the Social History Form has been initiated by the end of the first day of admission.

3. As soon as it becomes clear that either local authority or community nursing services are currently being provided on a regular basis, these agencies are notified of the admission. This should occur within 24 hours of admission or if at the weekend, as soon as the offices open.

4. The Hospital Admissions Office must send notification of the patient's admission to their GP (General Practitioner) or Health Centre as soon as possible, on the day after admission.

5. For patients living alone at the time of admission, the nurse in charge should ensure that:
   (a) a set of house keys has been located and kept either with the patient or in a safe place;
   (b) arrangements are made through friends/neighbours/ relatives to look after the accommodation, that any pets are cared for, and if not, then the Social Services are notified immediately;
   (c) any documents or valuables are itemized and kept with the patient or in the security department.

6. Any information coming in about a patient from a relative/ friend/neighbour is taken and recorded by nursing staff. All relevant information on the social circumstances of the patient should be collected, and sought if not offered, from relevant agencies by the time of the first planning meeting after admission.

7. At the planning meeting, a provisional plan is made for:
   (a) likely treatment;
   (b) likely length of stay;
   (c) the direction of discharge (e.g. own home, convalescence, extended care facility);
   (d) the patient's need for care at point of discharge;
   (e) any agencies which might offer care.

8. The plan is reviewed at each planning meeting subsequently and, as the patient returns to fitness, action is delegated to alert and involve relatives/friends of the patient and agencies as appropriate.
   The patient's consent is required prior to notifying any outside agencies of any of the patient's medical details. In the event that the patient does not consent, then it should be carefully explained to the patient that community services cannot be adequately arranged.

Representatives of all community agencies involved should be invited to planning meetings.

9. The decision on an appropriate avenue for discharge is made by the planning team in consultation with the patient and their family and friends.

10. All action necessary to prepare the patient and the home environment is instigated by the planning meeting. The views of the community agencies/family and friends should be given by the social work member of the team if the representatives are not able to attend themselves, or if not, by others who have met them. It is the responsibility of the social worker to see that these views are represented in some way at the planning meetings.

11. For patients being discharged to convalescence or extended care facilities, the date is set by the receiving facility. It must be clear that the hospital will readmit the patient if convalescence breaks down prior to his or her return home date.

12. If the patient is to return directly home and needs support, referrals should be made at least two weeks in advance of any likely discharge date to the relevant agency. This should be conducted in terms of a request for assessment of the patient whilst in hospital, i.e. before the next planning meeting. At the planning meeting, a date is fixed, having regard to service provisions, and all relevant agencies are notified of the decision on the same day.

13. The date of the discharge, if it involves community services, should be fixed at least one week in advance, and if possible, at the penultimate planning meeting, so that the final planning meeting confirms all arrangements.

14. As soon as the date of the discharge is set, all relevant parties are notified, including transportation services, if required.

15. The decision as to who notifies whom is made at the planning meeting.

16. During the last week in hospital, the patient should be visited by representatives of any agencies providing community care, and preferably by the individual carer.

17. Prior to discharge, each patient should receive written confirmation, on one document, of the dates and times of relevant visits to them by community services.

18. Before the patient leaves the ward, it is the responsibility of the nurse in charge on that day to ensure that:
    (a) the patient has all necessary drugs and dressings and has been instructed (preferably by a pharmacist) how to use them;
    (b) the patient has all valuables and effects held by the hospital given to them or their escort;

Table 11.1 Discharge policy

Aims

1. The safe discharge of all adults to situations where:
    - (a) their treatment and recovery will be continuous with that given in hospital
    - (b) their immediate needs for warmth, food and relief from pain are met
    - (c) they have shelter and are safe from molestation
2. The implementation of procedures for safe discharges for adults, and the monitoring of practices and progress
3. Close cooperation with Local Authority (Municipal) Services
4. Coordination of effort between hospital and community-based health care professionals
5. Establishing effective lines of communication with all parties involved

Objectives commensurate with these aims are to ensure that:

1. Each individual patient receives the care and attention necessary without having to compete with others
2. Where a patient is found to need nursing care, he or she will not be discharged unless there is suitable provision
3. All vulnerable patients (and those living alone) have someone to see them into their home
4. Planning for discharge starts as soon as possible (preferably before admission)
5. The handover of the care of the patient from hospital to the community should provide for continuous cover for the patient

Planning process

1. Weekly planning meetings are held by the ward team to coordinate and take responsibility for the recovery and safe discharge of all patients. It is essential that relevant community nursing staff attend these meetings
2. The planning meeting will assess the ability of the patient to manage the situation which will be encountered on discharge and advise the responsible physician accordingly
3. The planning meeting will decide which pre-discharge preparations are required and the Ward Sister (Head Nurse) is responsible for seeing that these preparations are put into effect and for setting a target date for the patient's discharge
4. The responsibility for successful discharge shall fall to the nurse in charge of the ward at the time of the patient's discharge. This nurse will have the authority to cancel the discharge if the arrangements agreed by the planning meeting are not yet completed
5. The discharge is not effective until the persons/agencies in the community have taken over any of the caring duties deemed necessary, and until that time, responsibility for the patient's continuing care shall remain with the hospital

6. Responsibility for medical cover must be transferred to the patient's general practitioner (family doctor) in advance of the patient's discharge
7. It is the responsibility of the Ward Sister to see that all parties concerned have been informed of the patient's discharge by the end of the discharge day

---

(c) they have access to their accommodation;
(d) there is someone to see them inside safely (other than transportation personnel);
(e) the patient is equipped with a written document of agencies who will be visiting him or her, with dates and times;
(f) where relevant, a letter for the receiving nursing advisor accompanies the patient;
(g) the patient has adequate supplies of food to last them until the next visit by someone providing a shopping service where needed;
(h) power, heating and water supplies in the accommodation are fully operational;
(i) the patient has enough money for essential needs to last him or her until the next day when banks/post offices are open;
(j) all relevant agencies have been fully informed;
(k) the patient is fully informed;
(l) all equipment and adaptations have been provided.
19. Responsibility for the care of the patient is transferred to the escort and then to the person settling the patient into the home. That person ensures that all items in 18 above, except (j), are correct before leaving the patient.
20. The escort or the receiver of the patient should take responsibility for notifying the discharging ward immediately of any deficiencies in the provision.
21. The patient can be said to have been safely discharged only when comfortably settled, with immediate needs for food, warmth and relief from pain met, and there is a comprehensive plan for the continuing care of that individual within the community, understood by all parties.

Discharge against medical advice

Attempts should be made to dissuade patients from taking their own discharge against medical advice. The patient may agree to see a counsellor or psychiatrist prior to leaving and if so, this should be facilitated. In every case, the patient is told (and this is documented in writing) that the health authority will accept no responsibility for the consequences of patients taking their own discharge and that community services cannot be guaranteed.

Community nursing personnel

1. Where a known patient is admitted to the hospital, the district nurse should notify the ward of the service being provided, including treatment given prior to admission. Where possible, this should be done by a visit to the ward.
2. If the patient is known to live alone, social services should be notified as soon as possible if arrangements are needed to protect the patient's home. Any action taken in this way is also to be notified to the ward.
3. When a known patient is to be discharged to the care of a district nurse, the district nurse should visit the hospital during the week preceding discharge in order to discuss the continuing care needs of the patient with both the ward nursing staff and the patient.
4. All home assessments should be carried out within 24 hours of the discharge.
5. The district nurse should notify the ward of the first day the visit can be made to the patient being discharged.

Local authority staff (municipal services)

1. Where a client of the social services is actively serviced by any of these sections:

Home Helps	Social Work	Community Social
Meals Service	Day Centre	Work
		Residential Homes

   and is known to have entered hospital, notice of the involvement is to be sent to the ward immediately.
2. Where the client lives alone, the agent of social services should ensure that arrangements have been made to protect the property.
3. The disclosure of any other personal details is only with the consent of the client.
4. The agent should telephone the ward to arrange a time to visit and to attend the next planning meeting. The agent should also notify the hospital social worker. Agents may decide it is appropriate for a hospital social worker to convey their views at the planning meeting and can negotiate with the hospital social work department for this to be done.
5. The agent should visit the client in hospital as soon as possible and

negotiate the release of information to the ward staff. This is then given to the nurse in charge.

6. During the patient's stay in hospital, any information or developments that occur in the home, including the care of any children, should be notified to the ward immediately.
7. All improvements to the home that are essential to the patient's safe return should be initiated as soon as they are identified and completed prior to the safe discharge of the client.
8. Adaptations in the home will be initiated by the hospital occupational therapy department and paid for by the local authority. Adaptations are to be completed prior to the safe discharge of the client.
9. As soon as a discharge date is foreseeable, the hospital will contact the community agencies for a service. Where the patient has not received a service within the last three months (including time in hospital), the agency will make an assessment of the level of need within one week of a request. Preferably this will entail a visit to the patient in hospital, and at the latest, a report within that week on the level of service that will be offered.
10. One week after the initial request for an assessment is made, a discharge date may be arranged depending on the findings and the views of the community.
11. Any objections or information should be communicated to the ward before or at the discharge planning meeting. For extremely dependent/handicapped clients, this may involve a separate conference at the hospital, which all agencies should endeavour to attend.
12. Where a patient goes to convalescence without being visited in hospital, the community agencies will have two weeks' notice of the return home date, and will assess on the first working day after return with a view to starting the service as soon as possible.
13. The patient will be visited within 24 hours of discharge by all agencies, or on the first working day where the full notice has been given.

District nursing service

Clearly enough district nurses in a health authority are required to be able to offer a nursing visit at any time of the day or night and at weekends. Many patients with AIDS can only be cared for safely in the community if they have access to round-the-clock nursing care. A central contact point which can identify and locate any district nurse in the area, 24 hours a day, is required. This involves clerical support and a paging system.

Home carers scheme

Within the group of Home Help employees, a team should be set up which can provide all that a caring relative might to a patient with AIDS living in the community. This scheme would require special training for these individuals to enable them to carry out special tasks as, for example, assistance with personal hygiene.

Discharge co-ordinator

The appointment of a discharge coordinator facilitates the safe and efficient discharge of patients to home and to community services. The discharge coordinator can assist in planning an unbroken chain of individualized patient care by facilitating effective communications between patients, relatives, friends, hospital and community agencies, by participating on a practical level as well as an educational and advisory level. They can also assist in the promotion of quality assurance regarding transfers between hospital and community.

Nursing care in the community

All members of the primary health care team may be involved in the care of clients with HIV-related illness, for example general practitioner, health visitor, district nurse, family planning nurse, school nurse, practice nurse and community psychiatric nurse. Clearly their involvement in the discharge planning process is essential if continuity of care is to be realized. Clients should be encouraged to give permission for their GP (General Practitioner) to be fully informed of their condition so that meaningful community nursing care can be assessed and planned with the support of the client's medical advisor. On occasion, clients refuse to give permission for their GP to be informed of their diagnosis, and although the client's wishes must be absolutely respected, this situation is fraught with real difficulties and the client should be explicitly made aware that there are potential problems involved. In these circumstances, district nurses will have to liaise with hospital medical staff in caring for these individuals. However, most GPs establish trusting relationships with their clients and it is becoming more unusual for patients to refuse permission for their GP to be informed of their medical condition.

Clients with AIDS and AIDS-related conditions can live safely with healthy members of the family in the community without any fear of HIV transmission from the client to family and friends. In advising clients with HIV infection, community nursing staff should take the following points into consideration.

Personal hygiene. Good general personal hygiene practices should be adopted. Razors, toothbrushes or other implements which could become contaminated with blood should not be shared. Sanitary towels must be disposed of in heavy-duty yellow plastic bags which can be discreetly collected and sent for incineration along with other contaminated wastes. Tampons may be flushed down the toilet. Individuals with HIV infection should wear gloves when cleaning fish bowls, bird cages, gardening and dealing with cat litter trays because of the risk of contamination with potential parasitic pathogens (e.g. *Toxoplasma gondii, Cryptococcus neoformans*).

General hygiene. Individuals with HIV infection can safely prepare, cook and serve food for others, observing usual standards of good hygiene (i.e. hands washed prior to food preparation and after handling any uncooked foods). Special crockery and cutlery is not necessary and all crockery and cutlery should be washed after use in hand hot water with a detergent (a disinfectant is not needed) and left to drip dry.

Linen visibly contaminated with blood, body fluids, excretions or secretions can be safely washed in a washing machine on the hot cycle. The hot cycle on standard washing machines exceeds the DH recommendations of 71°C (160°F) for not less than three minutes plus mixing time. The temperature and the addition of a detergent will inactivate any HIV and added disinfectants are not necessary. If the patient is too ill to do his or her own laundry, it can be done by a Home Help, friends or if necessary, arrangements can be made by the district nurse to have it processed at a local authority laundry. In this case, it is first placed in a water-soluble red plastic bag which is placed in a red nylon (or heavy-duty plastic) bag. In general, district nurses make arrangements with the environmental health department in their local authority to collect the laundry. This must be done discreetly; colour-coded bags of contaminated laundry or rubbish must not be left outside the patient's home, visible to neighbours and collection personnel must be well educated so that they do not arrive wearing bizarre protective clothing (which, of course, is not necessary). If this point is not attended to, inadvertent breaches of confidentiality might result with disastrous consequences for the client.

Individuals with HIV infection can use the same toilet and bath or shower as anyone else in the household; normal domestic cleaning is adequate after use (disinfectants are not necessary).

Clearly individuals with HIV infection may use, for example, the library, pub, restaurant, cinema, as any other member of the community might. There is no possibility of HIV transmission in public swimming baths[2].

In general, individuals with HIV infection should be encouraged to continue their usual employment and they may have to be discreet regarding informing their employer and fellow workmates of their medical condition.

Patient education. Health education designed to promote the primary prevention of others and secondary prevention for the client should be implemented. District nurses will need to discuss 'safer sex' practices with clients and leaflets are available from a variety of sources, for example the Terrence Higgins Trust and Health Education Authority. Individuals with HIV infection should be advised not to donate blood, tissues, organs, semen or carry donor cards. They should not breast-feed infants. Patient education is discussed in more detail in Chapter 12.

Dental treatment. Ideally clients who are infected with HIV should inform their dentist of this fact when presenting for treatment. However, this has often resulted in a refusal by a dentist to treat an infected individual. As all dentists have been advised by the DoH in the UK, and the CDC in the USA[3, 4], to observe **Universal Precautions** on all patients, all the time, regardless of what they know or do not know regarding their serological status for anti-HIV, it probably is in the client's best interest if they do not inform their dentist of their infectivity. This is an unfortunate state of affairs however it must be realized that dentists (and doctors) do not have the same ethical duty of care towards clients as professional nurses do and, can quite legally, refuse to treat (except in an emergency) individual patients.

The following points should be considered when assessing and planning care for clients in the community. It is essential that community nurses caring for patients with HIV infection are themselves free of any infectious illness (e.g. colds, herpes labialis) so as not to transmit any infections to the client. Good handwashing technique, prior to nursing the patient and on completion of nursing care, is required. Community nursing staff (and their managers) must know and understand the local operational policies and procedures for the community nursing care of clients with HIV-related illness. If no operational policies and procedures exist, they should be urgently prepared.

1. Community nurse managers should ensure that all equipment needed for the usual IC precautions is readily available to community nurses. This will include supplies of:
   - appropriate disinfectants (e.g. 'Presept' granules (NaDCC) or 'Virusorb' absorbent powder (chlorine powder)) and

NaDCC ('Presept') disinfectant tablets. Disinfectants are chiefly needed to deal with spillages, which are not common
- plastic aprons
- effective, high filtration face masks (e.g. 'Vigilon' masks)
- disposable non-sterile rubber latex or good quality plastic gloves (of the correct size!)
- red plastic bags for contaminated linen, and, red nylon linen bags
- sharps container (e.g. 'Daniels Sharps Bins')
- eye protection device
- heavy-duty yellow plastic bags for contaminated rubbish
- paper towels
- antiseptic soap (e.g. 'Betadine Surgical Scrub' or 'Hibisol')
- incontinence pads, dressing packs, and other nursing equipment
- specimen labels (e.g. 'BioHazard' or 'Risk of Infection')

2. **Sharps.** Extreme caution must be taken when dealing with or disposing of needles and other sharp instruments. A suitable sharps container can be left in the client's home until it is two-thirds full, when it is sealed and arrangements are made to collect it for incineration. Small portable sharps containers are available (Daniels – 'Safe-T-Bin') which can be safely carried by the district nurse.

3. **Injections.** Community nurses must wear disposable gloves when giving injections or during venesection. Needles must never be recapped or reinserted into their original sheaths and the needle is not disengaged from the syringe prior to disposal, but is disposed of as a single unit into the sharps container. The only exception is after the collection of blood, the needle is carefully disengaged from the syringe (preferably with a needle holder) to avoid a microscopic aerosol contamination when the blood is injected into the specimen container. Vacuum collection devices (e.g. 'Vacutainers') are preferable to a syringe and needle for venesection.

4. **Inoculation accidents and mucosal contamination with blood.** Follow the procedure outlined in Chapter 8 (Table 8.7).

5. Any cuts or open lesions on the arms or hands of nursing personnel must be covered with a waterproof, occlusive plaster (tape). Nurses with eczema should not deliver care to any client, including those with known HIV infection.

6. No protective clothing or IC precautions are required to enter the client's home, for introductions (shaking his or her hand) or talking to the client.

7. If the client has restricted mobility and cannot use the toilet, a

bedside commode or 'chemical toilet' may be useful. Bed pans and urinals are carefully emptied into the toilet (avoiding splashing), rinsed and stored dry (i.e. they are not left soaking in a disinfectant). District nurses wear disposable gloves when handling bed pans and urinals and when dealing with incontinent clients. After flushing, it is not necessary to pour disinfectants into the toilet.

8. **Spillages.** Spillages of blood, or those body fluids listed in Chapter 8, Table 8.1 from any patient, including those known to be infected with HIV, are carefully covered with a suitable disinfectant, such as 'Presept' granules, left for 5–10 minutes and then carefully wiped up with disposable paper towels which are disposed of into a yellow plastic bag. Nurses wear gloves and a plastic apron when dealing with spillages. If spillages occur on carpets, they are carefully mopped up with paper towels and chlorine or NaDCC disinfectants are not used. After wiping up the spillage, the area of carpet can be cleaned with a detergent and hot soapy water.
   The client should be encouraged to maintain social relationships and not to become isolated. Family and friends frequently require reassurance regarding the infectious nature of the client's condition.

9. **Terminal care.** Many clients with HIV-related conditions will require terminal care at home. This is not always possible due to neurological dysfunction or lack of any non-nursing support from family or friends. However, the terminal care of clients with AIDS at home is otherwise much the same as it is for any other client. Attention to symptom control is paramount and this will require a twilight or night community nursing service.

10. **Death at home.** The usual last offices are carried out observing the same IC precautions which were in operation when the client was alive. Disposable gloves and aprons are worn by those performing last offices. Undertakers will bring a plastic cadaver bag and will put the body into it. Once the body is in the cadaver bag, transport personnel do not require any protective clothing to handle the body.

Specialist community nurses

It may be useful for Health Authorities to train and appoint a specialist district nurse (ideally, a community nurse teacher) to act as an expert resource for his or her colleagues. However, all community nurses must become expert in the care of clients with HIV infection and the unique issues involved in this disease. Community nurses are by the very virtue of their training clinical nurse specialists and it is not necessary to establish a further specialization within district nursing.

Summary

Operational policies must exist which allow community nurses the time to complete a home-care nursing assessment prior to the client's discharge from hospital. The actual delivery of nursing care to clients with an HIV-related illness in the home is exactly the same as that required for the nursing care of any seriously ill client. Because of the various opportunistic infections clients with AIDS may present with, additional IC precautions, beyond Universal Precautions, may be needed. Community nurses have an immense role to play in this epidemic – perhaps the most critical role of all. Every opportunity for health education must be embraced and with careful discharge planning, district nurses will be able to coordinate all the services clients require. These nurses are strategically placed to make a real impact on the quality of care required and evidence to date indicates they are responding to this challenge with their usual brand of improvization, courage and compassion.

References

1. Crowther, P.., Donnelly, D., Hill, P., *et al.* (1987). *Discharge from hospital*. A discussion document with reference to the Riverside (West) Health Authority (2 February)
2. Royal Society of Medicine (1987). Public Swimming Pools and AIDS. *The AIDS Letter*, 1 (4):8
3. DHSS (1986). Guidance for Surgeons, Anaesthetists, Dentists and their Teams in Dealing with Patients Infected with HTLV-III. *Acquired Immune Deficiency Syndrome AIDS, Booklet 3* (April), CMO (86)7:6
4. Centers for Disease Control (1987). Recommendations for Prevention of HIV Transmission in Health-Care Settings. *MMWR* (August 21), 36(2S):7–8S

12

The Nurse As A Health Educator

At the end of this chapter, the reader will:

[Short-term Goal] *Understand* the underlying principles and practice of patient education and *have an opportunity* to demonstrate the technical skills needed to effectively participate in primary, secondary and tertiary health promotion activities.

[Long-term Goal] Be *enabled* to practice the skills of health education and fulfill the educative role of the Professional Nurse.

[Objectives]
1. *Describe* a systematic model of health education appropriate for use in a clinical setting.
2. *Identify* the critical elements of:
   2.1 assessing learning needs
   2.2 planning an educational response
   2.3 implementing patient education encounters
   2.4 evaluating learning
3. *Demonstrate* practice techniques related to effective patient education.
4. *Discuss* obstacles to patient learning.
5. *Outline* a strategy for patient education activities in your own practice setting.

The concept of the nurse as a 'health educator' is implicit in the definition of nursing as described by Henderson[1] and explicit in the Philosophy for Nursing of the Riverside Health Authority[2]. In the United Kingdom, 'Project 2000' programmes which prepare individuals to become Registered Professional Nurses stress the importance of ensuring that learners acquire skills in relation to the "identification of health related learning needs of patients and clients, families and friends and to participate in health promotion[3]." Today, in the 'age of AIDS,' the role of the nurse in primary, secondary and tertiary prevention is paramount. This chapter is designed to illustrate effective patient/client education techniques which nurses can use as 'educators for health' in primary, secondary and tertiary prevention roles (Fig. 12.1).

There are various models of health education available, all having relevance and uses with different individuals, cultures and situations. Although no single model of health education is always ideal in the variety of situations found in clinical practice, probably the most useful for nurses is an eclectic 'educational model' (Fig. 12.2). This is based on the belief that *health behaviour is a product of prior learning and that this behaviour can be changed by educational processes.* In this model, the nurse acts as a teacher and the patient/client accepts the role of the learner. This approach has been labelled 'teaching for health' and has been extensively described by Coutts and Hardy[4] [*see* Fig. 12.3]. Inherent in an educational model is the ability of the nurse to **assess** the learning needs of patients/clients and relatives and potential learning opportunities available, **plan** patient/client education programmes, **implement** appropriate teaching methods and techniques which promote health and **evaluate** the effectiveness of the patient/client educational encounters.

Assessing Learning Needs: (Fig. 12.4) Different individuals have

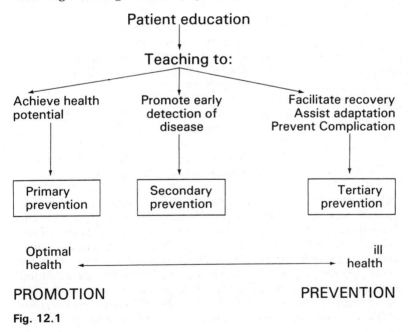

Fig. 12.1

Assess learning needs/potential
learning opportunities

Plan education programmes

Implement appropriate teaching

Evaluate effectiveness of encounter

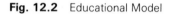

Fig. 12.2   Educational Model

informing (giving information)
advising
helping with the acquisition of skills
assisting with the process of clarifying beliefs, feelings and values
enabling the adaptation of lifestyle
promoting change in the structures and organisations which influence
   health status
providing a model of values and behaviour related to health

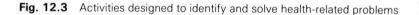
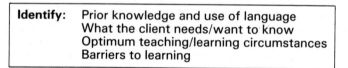

Fig. 12.3   Activities designed to identify and solve health-related problems

Identify: Prior knowledge and use of language
What the client needs/want to know
Optimum teaching/learning circumstances
Barriers to learning

Fig. 12.4   Assessing Learning Needs

different learning needs, often based on their intelligence, education,
social and cultural background. The patient/client's perception of
what they need to know is often different to that of the nurse. The best
way to establish what a patient/client needs to know is just to ask
him/her, e.g. 'what is your understanding of high risk sexual behaviour?' or 'can you explain to me how your discharge medications are
to be taken?' This allows the nurse an opportunity to ascertain prior
knowledge and to assess the language (i.e., the words) the patient uses
to communicate with and to describe behaviour. This will assist in
determining what learning deficits exist and inform as to how much the
patient/client wants, needs (and is able) to learn. It is essential to
provide privacy and time to adequately define learning needs and to

Differences between teacher & client in cultural, social & educational background & differences in primary language

Different values, sex, sexual orientation, religion, beliefs

The client is not receptive due to:-
confusion
pain
depression
fatigue
anxiety

The client has received contradictory messages from other sources

Faults in the teaching plan/technique: lack of privacy, time, lack of competence and/or confidence of teacher

Language used is not understood by client or client's language is not understood by the nurse

Fig. 12.5   Barriers to Effective Communications

give the patient/client permission and opportunity to ask questions. It is axiomatic that the nurse must know the patient and his individual circumstances, have clinical confidence and competence to engage in an educational encounter in relation to the specific issue being discussed and is comfortable in using language familiar to the patient.

During this phase, it is important to assess the optimum circumstances in which effective patient education encounters can be initiated. Learning can only occur when the individual is ready to learn. Barriers to learning include pain, high levels of anxiety and denial (Fig. 12.5)

Planning an educational response: Planning a patient education activity takes into account the educational technique to be used, the timing of the activity and the end product (i.e., the goals) (Fig. 12.6). Goals are sometimes referred to as 'Aims' and are defined as *broad, general statements of goal direction, which contains reference to the worthwhileness of achieving it*[5]. Just as the assessment phase involves the patient, so to must the planning stage (to the extent his/her clinical condition permits). The goals/aims of the activity must be negotiated with the patient. This involves asking the patient what he/she wants to know, what they think they should know or offering possible learning options. In addressing learning needs, the client and the nurse should negotiate

Negotiate: Goals (Aims), i.e.,   broad, general statements of
goal direction, which contain
references to the
worthwhileness of achieving it.

Short-term Goal(s) & Long-Term Goal(s), i.e.,

what the client **will be able to do** as a result of the teaching/
learning encounter

e.g. Teaching Session: Safer Sexual Behaviour
Short-term goal: ''at the end of this session, the
client will *understand* the sexual
means of HIV transmission''
Long-term goal   ''at the end of this session(s), the
client will be *enabled* to adopt a
safer means of expressing his/her
sexuality in order to prevent
secondary infectious disease
acquisition & transmission of HIV to
others

Fig. 12.6   Planning an Educational Response

Specify: Objectives, i.e., carefully constructed statements
which indicate with precision what
the client will be able to do at the
end of the teaching/learning session

Objectives are derived from the goals

Fig. 12.7   Planning an Educational Response

both short-term and long-term goals (i.e., what the client will be able to
do or accomplish as a result, both in the short-term and in the longer-
term, of the educational encounter). For example, a *short-term goal*
that might be negotiated with a client in reference to safer sexual
behaviour might be that at the end of the session, the client would
understand the sexual means of HIV transmission. The *long-term goal*
might be that the client would be enabled to adopt safer ways of
expressing his/her sexuality in order to prevent secondary infectious
disease acquisition and transmission of HIV to another individual.

Short-Term Goal:	''at the end of this session, the client will understand the sexual means of HIV transmission''
Objectives:	''at the end of this session, the client will:

1. *List* the body fluids which may transmit HIV
2. *Describe* the types of sexual behaviour which will facilitate HIV transmission
3. *Discuss* ways in which he/she can adopt a safer form of sexual expression
4. *Identify* potential problems with partner(s) in changing to a safer sexual life style
5. *Demonstrate* (on an antomical model) the correct use of a rubber condom

Objectives have a built-in evaluation facility

Fig. 12.8   Teaching Session: Safer Sexual Behaviour

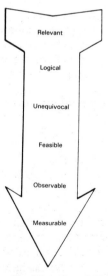

Relevant

Logical

Unequivocal

Feasible

Observable

Measurable

Fig. 12.9   Qualities of a Specific Educational Objective

Once the goals have been negotiated, the intended learning outcomes (i.e., objectives) of the session are derived and can be specified (Fig. 12.7). *Objectives are carefully constructed statements which indicate with precision what the client will be able to do at the end of a teaching/learning session.* Objectives are written for and directed at the client and are action verb statements, i.e., they describe what behaviour the client will be able to achieve at the end of the session. For example, a specific objective might be 'at the end of this session, the client will be able to *describe* high risk sexual behaviours,' or 'with the use of a anatomical model, *demonstrate* the correct use of a condom' (Fig. 12.8). Each action verb used in objective statements describe a specific behaviour which is observable, measurable, logical, feasible, unequivocal and relevant (Fig. 12.9). The 'goals and objectives' at the beginning of this chapter offer another example of setting the intended learning outcomes of a planned educational initiative. Objectives are usually constructed to describe *cognitive* (i.e., thinking) and *psycho-motor skills* which will result from the teaching/learning process and as such, have a built-in evaluation facility. Objectives can also be directed at different cognitive levels, for example knowledge, comprehension, application, analysis, synthesis and evaluation. More difficult to evaluate, but also useful, are objectives which can be directed towards *affective* (i.e., valuing, feeling and attitude formation) domains (Fig. 12.10).

Goals and specific objectives are much like a brick wall. The wall itself is the goal (or aim) and each individual brick is an objective. Initially, the short-term and long-term goals, along with the specific objectives should be written down by the nurse in order to have a check-list to evaluate the degree of learning that has taken place after the

Cognitive	– process of thinking, of acquiring information & working with it
Affective	– incorporates values, attitudes beliefs & feelings which create idiosyncratic reactions. Has important motivation influences
Psycho-motor	– acquisition of a motor skill perfected throughout practice

Fig. 12.10 Types and Levels of Learning

encounter(s). Once the goals and objectives have been negotiated and specified, the nurse can select the appropriate teaching method. In patient education encounters, the most common methods used are *one-to-one discussions* in which the current knowledge, attitudes and behaviour of the client are assessed, clarifying or giving additional information or facilitating the development of skills (e.g. decision-making, psycho-motor, assertion skills, etc.). *Demonstrations* are also a method commonly used in patient education encounters (e.g. the use of camouflage make-up, using a condom). In the planning stage, any teaching equipment/aids, written guidelines or literature may also be considered. A simple and brief teaching plan should be constructed, which includes the goals and objectives of the session, the step-by-step implementation of the session and a brief evaluation of what learning took place. This teaching plan should form part of the documentation of care given in the nursing care plan.

Preparing a teaching plan: This plan should firstly consider the teaching method or techniques which seem best suited to achieve the goals negotiated with the patient/client. The first consideration is that the method or technique choosen allows for maximum involvement of the patient. This is facilitated by using effective non-verbal communication skills, building into the plan opportunities for frequent question and answer periods and to be involved in the verbal summary of the session. If the goal is directed towards enabling the acquisition of a psycho-motor skills (e.g. preparing intravenous medication for administration through a Hickman catheter), then the teaching plan should include an opportunity for *immediate supervised practice* following the demonstration.

The teaching plan should include a *short introduction*, the *main body* of the teaching material, a *summary* and a *question and answer* period (Fig. 12.11).

The introduction should include the goals (both short-term and long-term) and objectives of the session and should establish the importance of the session.

The material in the main body of the session should follow a logical sequence. As the nurse will have already established, during the assessment period, the prior knowledge of the patient, the teaching session should be directed at: working from the known to the unknown, from familiar to unfamiliar knowledge and concepts, from basic to advanced material, from questions to answers and from identified problems to solutions.

The summary should include a review of the original goals and objectives of the session and repeat the important points made during the main body of the talk.

Finally, questions and answers will help clarify information for the

Prepare:	**Teaching Plan**
	Introduction: Establish significance of session and clarify goals and objectives
	Main Body: Work from: Known to the unknown Familiar to the unfamiliar Knowledge to concepts Basic to advanced Questions to answers Problems to solutions
	Summary: Review goals & objectives Repeat important points
	Questions and Answers Clarify information Primary evaluation opportunity

Fig. 12.11   Planning an Educational Response

patient/client and allow for the first evaluation of the achievement (or non-achievement) of the short term goal(s).

Implementing patient education: Effective teaching requires effective communication skills, both verbal and non-verbal. Non-verbal communications (i.e., body language) are critical and include (Fig. 12.12).

Proximity, i.e., how close you are to the client. Individuals with HIV infection and AIDS often feel isolated and stigmatised and effective teaching means being close to the client, without invading their personal space. Teaching sessions should not be conducted from the foot of the bed or with the nurse standing over a patient lying in bed. Either both the nurse and the patient are sitting in chairs relatively close

Effective use of Body Language, e.g. proximity, touching, facial expressions, eye contact, posture, hand and head movements, orientation, physical appearance.

Fig. 12.12   Implementing Patient Education

to each other, or if the patient is in bed, the nurse is sitting near the patient's head.

Body Contact, i.e., touching. Although in formal teaching practice, body contact is not generally useful, in patient education, especially with an individual who has HIV-related conditions, touching can convey many effective messages, such as 'I care and I'm here for you' and 'I'm not afraid.' Touching has to be done sensitively and is often over-done, resulting in counter-productive reactions.

Facial Expressions convey a wealth of information and a 'dead-pan,' non-reactive facial expression is not useful. Nurses who practice good listening skills, as described by Ewles and Simnett (6) and who are enthusiastic and responsive to the client and their material, convey a real sense of sincerity.

Eye contact should be scanning in nature, not staring which would make the client feel uncomfortable. Good, intermittent eye contact is needed, from speaker to listener during educational encounters. Generally, the listener (be it the nurse or the client) will look directly (straight in the eyes) at the speaker. If this doesn't happen, it is an indication that for one reason or another, the listener may not be paying attention to the speaker. There may be many reasons (e.g. material is uncomfortable to the listener, the language used is not being understood, the client is in pain, etc.) and this is an important clue to the speaker.

Posture sends messages to both the health educator and client. Sitting with arms crossed and fists clenched may signal significant anxiety which precludes learning until the underlying cause of the anxiety is addressed.

Many other aspects of body language, e.g. hand and head movements, orientation (i.e., the layout of the room), physical appearance (e.g. uniform versus casual/professional clothes) and movements are all important in teaching and learning, especially in semi-formal and formal teaching environments. Maintaining good **listening skills** is an essential ingredient at all stages of the teaching process (Fig. 12.13). It is

---

expressive concentration, inviting the client to talk,
giving attention, encouraging, reflecting
meanings/feelings, paraphrasing, summing up.

Fig. 12.13   Effective use of Listening Skills

an *active* process which helps the client talk, ask questions and partici-pate in the learning process. Effective listening assists in clarifying the client's attitudes, beliefs and values. These skills include:

Expressive concentration on what the speaker is saying. This involves the non-verbal body language skills discussed previously, e.g. good eye contact, reactive facial expressions, posture and head movements (e.g., nodding in understanding), etc.

Inviting the client to talk, e.g. "how do you feel about what I've just said" or "how can you use the information we've discussed this morning?"

Being attentive, e.g. maintaining steady eye contact, making neutral noises such as "I see . . ." or "yes . . .," etc.

Paraphrasing involves re-stating the essential aspects of what the client is saying, e.g. "so, you're worried your partner will be put off having sex if you wear a rubber condom."

Reflecting feelings verbally mirrors back to the client feelings you perceive he/she is communicating, e.g. "you are clearly worried about how your parents will react to the news that you are gay."

Reflecting meanings adds content to feelings, e.g. "you are frightened because you are scheduled for a bronchoscopy this afternoon."

Summarising is useful in clarifying the material the client is giving you and should be used throughout active listening, not just at the end of the teaching session. Summarising involves making brief statements which reflects the salient points the client has made, e.g., "so far, it seems that what you are saying is. . . ."

In implementing the main body of the teaching session, the following principles are useful to consider (Fig. 12.14):

Time: Negotiate with the patient when the session will start and ensure that you are there on time. Keep the session brief. It is far better to have several brief sessions which the client can concentrate on, rather than a long, tiring session. People who are ill or worried or who have some degree of sub-clinical cognitive dysfunction as a result of HIV infection, often find it difficult to concentrate for more than fifteen or twenty minutes at a time.

Principles of Implementation

Start on agreed time and keep session brief
(15–20 minutes)
State the most important things first
Repeat and stress critical points
Give clear, precise and specific advice
Avoid using jargon
Give written information

Fig. 12.14 Implementing Patient Education

State the most important things first. Clients will often remember the first things said and objectives should be prioritised so that critical points are discussed first.

Repeat and stress critical points. Without being tedious, it is important to repeat and re-emphasise critical points, e.g., "the most important aspect in adopting safer sexual behaviour is to avoid penetrative sex without using a rubber condom."

Give clear, precise and specific advice. For example, "You will be taking Foscarnet through your Hickman catheter every day, except Saturday and Sunday. It is important that you adjust your administration set so that the Foscarnet takes two hours to run it," *rather than* "take your Foscarnet five days a week and run it in slowly."

Avoid using jargon and long words and sentences. It may be appropriate to use medical terminology in order to help the client communicate easily with other health care professionals, but if medical terminology is used, it must be carefully explained to the client and, during the evaluation stage, any terminology used must be re-checked to ensure the client actually understands it.

Give written information to the client and go through the information with him/her. It is sometimes possible to have the client write down the important points covered and as this actively involves the client in the learning process, can be useful. Obviously having the client take dictation is *not* useful.

If the learning goals include teaching a psycho-motor skill, then the

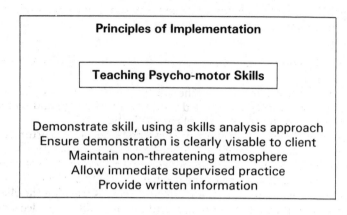

Fig. 12.15   Implementing Patient Education

following essential principles must be included in the teaching plan (Fig. 12.15).

Demonstrate the skill. In doing so, it is important that all the equipment (if any) used is prepared and at hand and that the demonstration is easily visible to the client. Part of the demonstration should include a skills analysis, i.e., the components of the skill are broken down into stages, starting with component 1, then component 2 and so on until the totality of the components equal the skill being taught. For example, if the client is being taught to administer his own aerosolised pentamidine, the skills analysis might be:

1. Attach a needle to 10 ml. syringe.
2. Wipe off the rubber top of the vial of bacteriostatic water with an alcohol swab and let dry.
3. Uncap the needle-guard from the needle.
4. Insert the needle into the rubber top of the vial of water.
5. Pull back on the plunger of the syringe and draw up 6 ml. of water.
6. Carefully with-draw the needle and syringe from the vial of water.
7. Put the needle guard back on the needle.
8. Wipe off the rubber top of the lypophilised pentamidine with an alcohol swab and let dry.
9. Take the needle-guard back off the needle.
10. Insert the needle into the rubber top of the pentamidine vial and inject the 6 ml. of water.
11. Withdraw the needle and syringe and cover the needle again with the needle-guard.

12. Shake the vial of pentamidine and water until the pentamidine is fully dissolved.
13. Etc.

Full, simple written instructions as per the skills analysis should be left with the client.

During the learning session, the teacher needs to ensure that the atmosphere is friendly and relaxed (i.e., non-threatening) and remain enthusiastic in order to keep the client motivated.

Following the demonstration, it is essential that an opportunity is built into the learning session for immediate supervised practice by the client so that the skills can be consolidated and re-enforced. This is also part of the evaluation stage of the teaching/learning process.

If part of the learning goals are directed towards teaching the client both affective (feeling) and cognitive (thinking) skills, e.g. decision-making skills, the following points are important (Fig. 12.16):

Help the client **define the problem**, e.g., "I can't find a way to tell my wife I'm infected with HIV."

Clarify the clients goals, e.g. "I don't want to infect my wife."

Help the client **define alternative methods** of achieving the goal, e.g. "Maybe the Doctor should tell her," or "I won't tell her but I'll only have safer sex with her in the future."

Help the client **identify the advantages and disadvantages** of each method, e.g. "If I don't tell her myself, she won't trust or respect me in the future." Let the client **decide** which is the best course of action, based on the above and discuss with the patient his/her **perception of the likely results** of that decision.

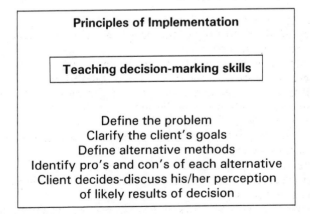

Principles of Implementation

Teaching decision-marking skills

Define the problem
Clarify the client's goals
Define alternative methods
Identify pro's and con's of each alternative
Client decides-discuss his/her perception
of likely results of decision

Fig. 12.16   Implementing Patient Education

Finally, in implementing planned teaching, **barriers to effective communication** should be identified and addressed, as discussed previously (Fig. 12.5).

Evaluating the teaching session: After summarising the main points of the session and answering the clients questions, the short-term goals and specific learning objectives are reviewed with the client and an evaluation assessment is made, i.e., the client did or did not achieve the learning objectives and the short-term goal. The long-term goals are evaluated at future teaching/learning sessions. The nurse should re-visit the client the next day, if possible, to re-check the evaluation assessment and to answer any further questions the client might have. **On-going assessment** will identify further learning needs and the process described in this chapter is repeated (Fig. 12.17).

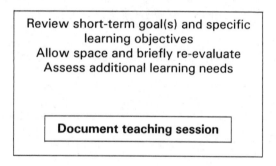

Fig. 12.17   Evaluating Teaching Session

Documentation of teaching: the teaching plan is entered into the client's notes and the teaching/learning session is documented in the Nursing Care Plan.

References

1.   Henderson, V. (1964). *Basic Principles of Nursing Care*, International Council of Nurses, Geneva
2.   Riverside Health Authority (1990). *Philosophy For Nursing*, 2nd edition, London
3.   Ridley, N. (1989). *The Nurses, Midwives and Health Visitors (Registered Fever Nurses Amendment Rules and Training Amendment Rules) Approval Order 1989*, Statutory Instruments, United Kingdom
4.   Coutts, L.C. and Hardy, L.K. (1985). *Teaching For Health; The Nurse as Health Educator*, Churchill Livingstone, London

5. Quinn, F.M. (1988). *The Principles and Practice of Nurse Education*, 2nd ed., Croom Helm, London
6. Ewles, L. & Simnett, I. (1985). *Promoting Health: A Practical Guide to Health Education*, John Wiley & Sons, Chichester, U.K.

13

The Management of Strategic Nursing Care: The 'Riverside Model'

The efficient delivery of individualized patient care requires informed, perceptive nursing management. The failure to develop competent and compassionate management services results in a breakdown of direct patient care, confusion and low morale among nursing staff, distress and isolation for the patient and a negative image of the hospital. Most metropolitan hospitals now have some experience in caring for patients suffering from HIV-related disease. In the beginning of the epidemic, a general commonality in problems and issues emerged. A core of expertise has now developed which other hospitals can use to avoid the early problems associated with the admission of a patient with AIDS.

Coordination of nursing care

Nursing management should initiate the formation of an 'AIDS coordinating committee', which should have broad educational and supportive responsibilities. The committee should be composed of both experts and non-experts and be representative of the hospital community. A typical coordinating committee might have the following membership:

Experts
infection control nurse
microbiologist
clinical nurse specialist
    (medical/oncology nursing)
dietitian
physician
clinical psychologist
clinical nurse specialist
    (psychiatric nursing)
nurse educationalists
social worker/health adviser
community nurse

Non-Experts
key Trade Union representatives
hospital chaplain
representative from domestic/
    housekeeping services
representative from transport/
    portering services
senior nurse – occupational
    health services
unit general manager or deputy
senior nurse manager

The committee must have visible and aggressive support from both nursing and hospital management and from experts within the hospital. The coordinating committee should have three major areas of responsibilities.

1. The formation and adoption of **Universal IC Precautions** as well as the monitoring of their implementation.
2. Planning and implementing in-service education and training programmes for all grades of staff.
3. Advising general management on policy and long-term planning for patients with HIV-related illnesses.

Hospitals which currently have little experience in caring for patients with HIV-related illnesses should form a coordinating committee and initiate planning prior to admitting their first patient. It is inconceivable that any general hospital will not be responsible for caring for these patients in the future. Planning now will dissipate initial anxiety and confusion.

In-service education

Hospitals which have developed pro-active in-service educational programmes for their staff have been the most successful in minimizing anxiety and disruption when a patient with HIV disease is admitted. In-service education should commence with orientation/induction of new staff and be on-going. A combination of various formats is the most useful approach, including workshops, seminars, study days and ward-based discussions and tutorials. Specialist nurse teachers and the infection control nurse are ideally placed to implement educational programmes, advised by the AIDS coordinating committee. A study day once a year on 'AIDS' is not adequate to deal with the new problems and issues posed by the admission of patients with HIV disease.

Infection control nurse

If not already in post, the recruitment of a clinical nurse specialist in infection control is absolutely essential. Comprehensive, competent and safe patient care, both in hospital and at home, cannot be ensured without the support and advice of this specialist. With the advent of HIV disease, it would seem impossible to cope without the guidance of an IC nurse.

Conditions of employment

Contracts of employment for all health care workers must clearly preclude the withdrawal of care from any patient, regardless of age, sex, sexual orientation, race, religion or presenting illness. Nursing management must make it absolutely clear that nursing personnel do not have the right to choose whom they will or will not nurse. Management must be seen to be determined in enforcing this correct obligation of employment. Staff who are reluctant to care for a patient should be counselled and given additional in-service training. If their reluctance persists, they should be dismissed. Quality assurance strategies should be designed to ensure that patients are not suffering as a result of ignorance, prejudice or unethical and judgemental attitudes projected onto them by health care workers.

Dedicated wards and clinics

Metropolitan hospitals experiencing significant admissions of patients with HIV-related disease should consider the creation of dedicated units. The advantages of these units include:

1. Nursing care can be 'state of the art' and specialized care strategies can be developed to meet the complex psycho-social-medical issues seen in these patients.
2. Many patients with HIV-related illness prefer being cared for in a dedicated unit.
3. Motivated, concerned staff, comfortable with their own sexuality, can be recruited to these units and given additional specialist training. They will quickly gain knowledge of other available resources to enable them to formulate effective, early discharge planning.
4. Units are cost-effective and have a positive impact on bed availability. Effective discharge planning, centralized care and the identification of other resource issues can most efficiently take place within these units.
5. Units can attract additional funds from concerned groups in the community. There can be a positive public relations impact in their creation.
6. The body of knowledge upon which the profession is based can be increased by the expanding expertise acquired by the nursing staff in these units.
7. Personnel problems are minimized and hospitals which have created these units have experienced high staff morale and a correspondingly high level of patient satisfaction.

Dedicated units must have clear admission criteria and therapeutic objectives. Their existence does not mean that patients with AIDS will not be cared for in other areas of the hospital. Many patients with HIV-related illness do not require the intensive specialist care offered by dedicated units. Hospice and terminal care facilities should also be considered as dedicated units are generally designed as active treatment units. A dedicated unit will not be effective unless it is supported by a comprehensive dedicated out-patients clinic. These clinics should be able to screen patients, initiate diagnostic procedures and maintain out-patients by providing a range of services which include intravenous rehydration, blood transfusions and intravenous chemotherapy. Clinical nurse specialists need to be recruited and trained for dedicated clinics.

Counselling services and support groups

Hospitals need to develop comprehensive counselling services for patients with HIV-related disease. Although a multidisciplinary approach is needed for the complex problems seen in this disease, clinical psychologists have the most relevant skills and should lead the planning and implementation of these services. Health advisors, social workers and lay counsellors from concerned community groups (e.g. the Terrence Higgins Trust, London) can complement this service. If lay counsellors are used, facilities must be made available to them. Counselling is required at all stages of illness, from pre-screening counselling to bereavement support, both for in-patients and for out-patients. If a hospital is treating more than a few patients with HIV-related illnesses, a patient's 'Support Group' can be established. These groups are invaluable in providing space for venting emotions and offering mutual support. They can include both in-patients and out-patients. Hospitals which have large numbers of patients with AIDS and other HIV-related conditions often provide a sophisticated range of support groups. For example, patients with Kaposi's sarcoma may form one group as they have specific problems coping with alterations in body image which patients with opportunistic infections may not have. Intravenous substance abusers often respond only where other group members are also substance abusers. In addition, **staff support groups** are used to provide an opportunity for health care workers to explore their anxieties, frustrations and other related 'burn-out' problems. Support groups must be competently and sensitively led by a staff member especially trained for this role.

Confidentiality

Nursing management must be sensitive to the balance required between ensuring appropriate IC precautions and the need to ensure appropriate confidentiality. The implementation of **Universal Precautions** assists in maintaining confidentiality in that IC precautions are the same for all patients. Management must ensure that policies and procedures designed to ensure confidentiality are in place, understood by all staff and effectively monitored.

Public relations

Contact with the media presents both potential problems and opportunities for the hospital to assume a leadership role in health education. In dealing with the press, precise and honest information will diminish adverse publicity. It is useful if an expert and authoritative representative of the hospital staff is designated as the spokesperson for the hospital on all HIV-related issues. All hospital staff members should be required to coordinate all press communications through this individual. Maximum use should be made of written press releases when information is requested rather than verbal interviews, which are often 'reinterpreted' by the media. The overriding principle of public relations is the maintenance of patient confidentiality and dignity.

Employment of health care workers who are infected with HIV

Currently, many hospitals have experienced situations where a member of their staff has developed AIDS/ARC or is asymptomatically sero-positive for anti-HIV. This has included surgeons, dentists, nurses and ancillary staff. Excluding the rare documented incidents of gross needlestick injuries (discussed previously), these health care workers acquired HIV infection sexually. It seems probable that, in time, all sexually active individuals may be 'at risk' for HIV infection, including health care workers. Although the occupational risk of HIV transmission is minimal (or nil if the strategies outlined in this text are diligently followed), health care workers are members of the broader community and are as much at risk sexually as any other member of the community.

As it is inconceivable that routine screening for anti-HIV could ever be implemented, most individuals who are seropositive for anti-HIV will be unknown to the employing health authority. However, occasionally this information is made known to the health authority by the employee. More commonly, health care workers who develop clinical manifestations of HIV infection consult the occupational health services and, eventually, a diagnosis of AIDS or ARC is established. Early in the epidemic, some hospitals and health authorities reacted inappropriately to this situation by suspending or dismissing the employee on the grounds that they posed an unacceptable IC risk to the patients of the hospital. This is quite clearly wrong and several issues need to be addressed in establishing the correct response of an employing health authority faced with this increasingly common predicament.

1. The means of transmission for HIV are well established and well documented. Other than intravenous substance abuse, HIV infection is now almost exclusively a sexually transmitted disease. In a health care setting, person-to-person transmission of HIV from a health care worker to a patient, could probably only be achieved by sexual transmission. This would be an unusual, if not bizarre, event in hospital.

2. Consequently, there has only been one possible case of HIV transmission from an infected health care worker to a patient[1].

3. If a health care worker was infected with HIV, it would be essential that appropriate precautions were taken to eliminate any possibility of blood or body fluid contamination from the employee to a patient. This would include covering any cuts or abrasions on the hands with a waterproof dressing and wearing disposable gloves when engaging in direct patient care. Well established, appropriate precautions should also be taken to prevent transmission of any infection (e.g. herpes) to a patient. However, all of the precautions required amount to no more than good clinical practice, which all health care workers have a responsibility to maintain, *regardless* of their serological status for anti-HIV.

4. Health care workers involved in invasive procedures, such as surgery, midwifery or dentistry, may be thought to be more of a risk to patients if they are anti-HIV positive. Concern has been expressed that these health care workers should be reassigned to clinical duties, which do not involve invasive procedures. It is essential that management create a public stance on this issue and a model policy on the employment of HIV infected health care workers can be found in Appendix 7.

Patient's Bill of Rights

Nursing management should construct and communicate widely a philosophy of care with which both the patient and the nurse can identify. This philosophy should include a description of the patient's rights[2]. These rights should guarantee to all patients:

1. The right to quality health care in an atmosphere of human dignity without regard to age, ethnic or national origin, sex or sexual orientation, religion or presenting illness.

2. The right to receive emergency medical and surgical treatment.

3. The right to considerate, dignified and respectful care by all health

care workers, regardless of the patient's physical or emotional condition.

4. The right to be informed of the name, title and function of anyone involved in their care.
5. The right to receive upon request an explanation of their current medical condition in language that they can understand.
6. The right to give or decline true informed consent and to participate in the choice of treatment. If consent for treatment is not given, the right to be informed of the likely medical consequences of their action.
7. The right to privacy to an extent consistent with providing dignified medical and nursing care.
8. The right to confidentiality.
9. The right to be informed of and to participate in their discharge planning.
10. The right to refuse to participate in research projects.
11. The right to receive, upon request, a consultation and/or care and treatment from another appropriate physician on the staff other than the one assigned to them.
12. The right, both as a patient and as a citizen, free from restraint, interference, coercion, discrimination or reprisal, to voice grievances and complaints and to recommend changes in policies and services. This implies that patients have access upon request to senior nurse managers.
13. The right to expect visitors to be treated with courtesy and respect.

Resuscitation

In the current state of knowledge, patients with AIDS have a terminal illness. While it may be appropriate to offer ventilation and other life-support systems to patients with AIDS in the early stages, it is often not compassionate to do so in the end-stage of their illness. The patient must be involved in decisions regarding intensive care and resuscitation. It is the physician's primary responsibility to discuss this with the patient and to make the final decision. This decision must be clearly communicated to all health care workers directly involved with the care of the patient and is appropriately discussed at routine, multi-disciplinary case conferences.

Summary

The competent and compassionate management of nursing is as important as the direct nursing care delivered at the bedside. The issues discussed in this chapter must not come as a surprise to management.

Effective forward planning will facilitate the smooth running of the hospital and the delivery of quality care to all patients when patients with AIDS are admitted. Although each nurse is accountable for his or her own clinical and professional practice, nurse managers are individually accountable for providing adequate staffing levels, planning, guidance, formation of policies and procedures and for providing a philosophy of leadership, which promotes the high standards of care that all patients have a right to expect.

The 'Riverside Model'

Over ten years of experience in caring for an escalating number of individuals, both in hospital and in the community, has been gained by the Riverside Health Authority in London. This health authority embraces two large general hospitals (Charing Cross Hospital and the Westminster Hospital) a children's hospital (Westminster Children's Hospital), a major psychiatric hospital (Horton Hospital), comprehensive community and maternity services and a wide variety of health services available at smaller hospitals and clinics within the health authority. The Riverside Health Authority is currently caring for the majority of individuals with HIV-related illness in the UK. Comprehensive services are available for patients with AIDS/ARC within the authority and this includes dedicated in-patient and out-patient facilities. As there are such large numbers of patients with HIV-related conditions being cared for within the authority, it is recognized that patients with AIDS-related conditions will be nursed in all wards and departments of all hospitals and in the community.

The Nursing Advisory Committee

A vast amount of nursing, educational, medical and managerial expertise in caring for patients with HIV-related illnesses has been gained and an exciting model of nursing management has emerged, committed to ensuring that all patients/clients within the authority consistently receive meaningful, nonjudgemental, compassionate nursing care of the highest quality. The provision of this exemplary care is facilitated by the managerial structure of the health authority. Professional nursing advice to the authority is derived from the **Nursing Advisory Committee** (NAC). This committee is composed of Senior nurse managers and educationalists. The **AIDS Coordinating Group (Nursing)** was established to ensure that the NAC was fully informed on all the professional and managerial issues associated with HIV infection in order to advise general management appropriately.

The AIDS Coordinating Group (Nursing)

This subgroup of the NAC, composed of nursing experts in caring for patients/clients with HIV-related illnesses and senior nurse managers and educationalists, develops policies and procedures related to caring for patients with HIV infection and advises on the nursing education strategy for the Riverside College of Nursing. This strategy addresses the learning needs of both student nurses in pre-registration nursing education programmes and qualified nursing personnel (for examples of recommended educational strategies see Appendix 5). The AIDS Coordinating Group (Nursing) submits all draft policies and procedures and any further appropriate advice to the NAC for approval. Once approved by the NAC, they become part of the operational policies and procedures for nursing services within the authority.

Policies and procedures

It is essential that current infection control policies and procedures are formulated which take into account the changes in clinical practice required by the advent of HIV infection. Clearly, these policies and procedures must be based on current practice recommendations that *all* blood and body fluids from *all* patients in *all* health care settings must be regarded as potentially infectious and appropriate precautions taken. Senior Nurses for Infection Control and other experts advise the AIDS Coordinating Group (Nursing) on infection control procedures who then drafts appropriate policies and procedures for consideration by the **Infection Control Committee**. All infection control policies are reviewed on an annual basis and current, approved procedures are distributed to all service areas within the authority.

Philosophy for Nursing

It is essential that the mission of care within the nursing services is discussed, agreed and published and, further, is widely understood by all nursing employees within the authority. The **Philosophy for Nursing** acts as the essential underpinning for all specific policy statements by the NAC and is the professional reference for all subgroups of the NAC. The Philosophy for Nursing in the Riverside Health Authority[3] (see Appendix 6) is an exciting, dynamic concept which has guided nursing services in formulating the operational policies and procedures needed to effectively manage the nursing force within the authority as they confront the complexities of caring for large numbers of patients/clients with HIV-related illness. It is critical that nursing services within all health authorities define and describe their mission of care and that it is widely understood by all nursing service/education staff.

Specific policy statements

Nursing services should develop policies for their employees on the issues described in Table 13.1.

Table 13.1 Specific policy statements for nursing services

1. Universal Precautions
2. Duty of Care
3. Confidentiality
4. Consent for Serological Testing
5. Anonymous Prevalence Data Testing
6. Employment of Nurses who are Infected with HIV
7. Educational Strategy for HIV Infection

The policy statement on **Duty of Care** must be discussed (and documented as discussed) with all current nursing service employees and by all prospective candidates for nursing posts within the authority at interview.

Naturally, nurse managers must ensure that all approved policies and procedures are adhered to by all nursing service employees and initiate appropriate action should there be any inconsistencies in the implementation of the operational policies and procedures of the authority. These policies should be discussed at regular service unit meetings and at all orientation/induction programmes for newly joined nursing employees. They must be available for reference, along with the current infection control procedures, in all units of service.

The creation and ongoing monitoring of these operational policies and procedures increase the security of both staff and patients/clients and ensure that the nursing care being delivered is both current and safe. Without this type of forward planning, health authorities will find that the admission of individuals with HIV-related illnesses to their hospital and community services will create chaos and detract from the smooth running of health care services. Nurse managers have a professional obligation to ensure that nursing service employees are provided with appropriate guidance and support; these policies assist with this provision.

The current operational policy statements from the Nursing Advisory Committee of The Riverside Health Authority (i.e. the 'Riverside Model') are given in Appendix 7.

References

1. Centers for Disease Control (1990). Possible Transmission of Human Immunodeficiency Virus to a Patient during an invasive Dental Procedure, *MMWR* (July 27), **39**(29):489–93
2. New York City Health and Hospitals Corporation (1984). *Patient's Bill of Rights*, Office of Patient Relations, New York
3. Dorman, M., Forrest Riley, M., Jones, J. *et al.* (1990). *Philosophy for Nursing*, 2nd ed., The Riverside Health Authority, London

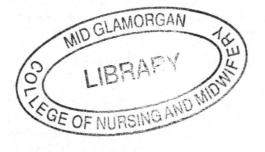

14

Nursing Issues related to the Medical Management of AIDS and HIV infection

With the recognition of HIV as the causative agent of AIDS, medical research has progressed rapidly on two fronts: towards the development of an effective treatment regime and the discovery and deployment of a biological vaccine.

Medical treatment

Current medical treatment is designed to slow viral replication and to treat and prevent episodes of opportunistic disease.

Antiviral agents

Antiviral therapy for HIV infection is based on the premise that continued viral replication is involved in both the pathogenesis and the progression of HIV disease and that suppression of HIV replication will reduce the direct and indirect effects of HIV infection.

The major drugs used today to suppress HIV replication are the dideoxynucleoside analogues, a group of drugs that inhibit the action of reverse transcriptase. The major drugs in this class are: **zidovudine (Retrovir), dideoxycytidine (ddC)** and **dideoxyinosine (ddI)**.

Retrovir (zidovudine), formerly known as **azidothymidine** (AZT), was discovered and introduced into the clinical care of patients with HIV-related illness by Burroughs-Wellcome in 1986. Retrovir is chemically similar to thymidine, a substance normally found in T4-helper cells. Thymidine is necessary for the reverse transcriptase in HIV to convert the viral RNA into viral DNA which is then incorporated into the host cell DNA (Fig. 14.1). By giving a thymidine analogue (i.e. 'fake' thymidine), the viral DNA formed (the 'transcript') is abnormal and cannot fully be integrated into the host cell DNA (Fig. 14.2). The result is that viral replication is halted, leading to clinical improvement in most patients. Patients feel well, gain weight, and clearance of chronic opportunistic infections is usually seen. The immune system has a chance of recovering and the numbers

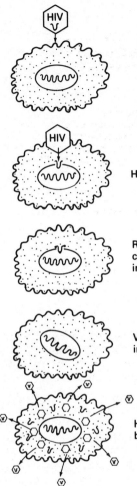

HIV RNA enters the T lymphocyte

Reverse transcriptase
converts viral RNA into viral DNA
in the presence of thymidine

Viral DNA becomes incorporated
into the host cell DNA

HIV infected T lymphocyte
becomes a viral factory

Fig. 14.1 HIV infection and replication

of circulating T4-helper cells increase. Although Retrovir is not a cure
for AIDS, it most definitely leads to a longer life of better quality.

Retrovir comes as 100 mg and 250 mg capsules and currently is
usually prescribed as 100 mg every four hours (600 mg total daily dose).
Previously, higher daily doses (e.g. 12–1500 mg total daily dose) had

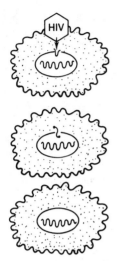

HIV infects the T lymphocyte
containing active zidovudine
(zidovudine triphosphate)

Reverse transcriptase
mistakes zidovudine triphosphate
for active thymidine (thymidine
triphosphate), zidovudine triphosphate
stops the formation of viral DNA

HIV cannot replicate

Fig. 14.2   Retrovir mode of action

been used but recent clinical trials have demonstrated a comparable
efficacy and less side effects using the lower treatment dose[1]. Retrovir
should be taken as an empty stomach.[2] Retrovir crosses the blood-
brain barrier and may improve or prevent the neurological effects of
HIV infection.

Retrovir is generally prescribed for individuals with HIV-related
illness but current discussions centre on the value of prescribing
Retrovir in asymptomatic infection. Retrovir must be taken for life and
is associated with significant side-effects in some individuals. These
side-effects include severe anaemia which usually occurs after four to
six weeks of therapy. Anaemia may require blood transfusions and
temporary cessation of Retrovir therapy. Leucopenia and neutropenia
may also be encountered and patients on Retrovir therapy should have
a full blood count every two weeks during the early stages of treatment
and then at monthly intervals. Other common side-effects include
nausea, rash, headache, fever and myalgia. Patients taking Retrovir
must not take paracetamol BP (acetamonophen USP) extensively, or
probenecid. Drugs which are known to be nephrotoxic, hepatotoxic or
myelosuppressive (e.g. **ganciclovir**) should not be taken while on
Retrovir therapy and patients should be cautioned about self-adminis-
tration of OTC (over-the-counter) drugs.

Other agents similar to Retrovir (i.e. **dideoxynucleoside analogues**) are currently in clinical trials. These include **dideoxycytidine (ddC)** and **dideoxyinosine (ddI)** and both may be combined with low dose Retrovir for a synergistic effect.

Antiretroviral agents other than zidovudine

There has been an explosion of scientific initiatives directed at exploiting differences between the biology of HIV and the host cells it infects. Although zidovudine is currently the only approved anti-retroviral agent for HIV infection, it is likely that during 1991/92 other agents will be available. Table 14.1 lists some of the newer agents which are now under investigation or in clinical trials.

Table 14.1   New antiretroviral agents

GLQ 233 (trichosanthin) Compound Q
antisense oligonucleotides
viral protease inhibitors
Ampligen
Hypericin
Dideoxycytidine (ddC)
Dideoxyinosine (ddI)
Castanospermine
n-butyl 1-deoxynojirimycin (n-butyl DNJ)
Pokeweed antiviral protein (PAP conjugates)

Prophylaxis of opportunistic infections

Although zidovudine therapy reduces the frequency and severity of opportunistic infections in individuals infected with HIV, patients who have T4 helper cell (CD4 + lymphocytes) counts below 200 mm3 (or CD4 + cells totalling less than 20% of total lymphocytes) are usually advised to initiate prophylaxis against the common opportunistic infections seen in AIDS. Common prophylaxis regimes which the nurse should be familiar with include:-

Pneumoycstis carinii pneumonia

The two most common approaches are[3]:

1. Oral **trimethoprim-sulfamethoxazole** (160 mg trimethoprim and 800 mg of sulfamethoxazole), i.e., two 'Septrin' or 'Bactrim' tablets, given twice daily.
2. **Aerosol pentamidine** given as 300 mg once monthly.

If the above two drugs are not tolerated, **dapsone**, with or without either **trimethoprim** or **pyrimethamine** may be prescribed. **Pyrimethamine-sulfadoxine ('Fansidar')** may also be used but seems less effective and more toxic than dapsone[4]. Fansidar may provoke a fatal **Stevens-Johnson syndrome** and should be used with caution.

All of the above drugs are associated with common side effects (discussed earlier) which nurses should anticipate during care evaluations.

Toxoplasma gondii Like most opportunistic infections seen in patients with AIDS, the cause is the activation of already present latent infection and some studies have found that 30–35 per cent of patients with AIDS have serological evidence of prior Toxoplasma gondii infection[5]. Patients infected with HIV should be serologically screened for T. gondii antibodies and if they are negative, patient education programmes should be implemented to teach the patient how to avoid acquiring T. gondii infection (Table 14.2).

Table 14.2 Primary Prevention of T. goodii Infection

Avoid eating under-cooked meats

Wash hands thoroughly after handling uncooked meat and avoid touching your mouth or eyes while handling uncooked meat

Thoroughly wash all kitchen surfaces which have come into contact with uncooked meat

Carefully wash all fruits and vegetables (especially lettuce!) prior to cooking or eating

Wear household gloves when dealing with cat litter trays and when working in the garden. Wash hands thoroughly after both activities.

If you have a cat litter tray, disinfect frequently

For patients who have serological evidence of past *T. gondii* infection or who have had *T. gondii* encephalitis, prophylaxis usually includes **pyrimethamine with sulfadizine**. **Clindamycin** may be used for those patients who cannot tolerate **sulfonamides** and may be given with **pyrimethamine**.

Candida infections (usually *C. albicans* but other species may be involved) are almost universal in patients with AIDS. **Fluconazole ('Diflucan')** is most commonly used for prophylaxis.

Cryptococcus neoformans – another fungal infection commonly seen in patients with AIDS may be prevented by the use of **fluoconzaole ('Diflucan')**.

Cytomegalovirus infections – either **ganciclovir** or **phosphonoformate ('Foscarnet')** are used for maintenance therapy. Primary prophylaxis is not practical.

Herpes simplex infection – **Acyclovir ('Zovirax')** is used for maintenance therapy but as acyclovir-resistant H. simplex infections can occur, it is not usually prescribed for primary prophylaxis.

Streptococcus pneumoniae – **polyvalent pneumococcal vaccination** should be offered to all HIV-infected individuals, early in the course of HIV infection (6).

Vaccination against HIV Infection

There is currently no biological vaccine available to protect against HIV infection, although impressive progress is being made to develop one. Several candidate vaccines have already been entered into clinical trials and it is possible that an effective vaccine may be developed during this decade.

Screening for Markers of HIV Infection

Following infection with HIV, several immunological reactions can be serologically observed (Fig. 14.3).

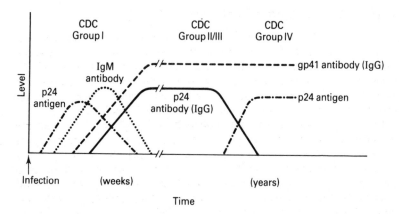

Fig. 14.3 Seriological markers of HIV infection

1. Within two to three weeks of infection, core antigens (p24) can be detected in the blood. A test to detect p24 antigens is often referred to as an 'antigen test.'
2. Shortly after the appearance of p24 antigens, IgM antibodies appear. These antibodies can be directed against the core (gag) proteins of the virus (i.e., p24, p18, p55) and the envelope (env) glycoproteins (i.e., gp120 and gp41). IgM antibodies to the virus are short-lived; IgM antibodies to p24 will be undetectable within three to four months, however IgM antibodies to gp41 can be detected for a longer period. **Their presence is a marker of acute (i.e., early) infection.**
3. Within three to six months, IgG antibodies to the transmembrane glycoprotein (gp41) start to appear. **These antibodies are long lasting and their detection is the basis of common serological screening tests.** IgG antibodies to other major structural gene products of HIV (i.e., gag and env proteins) are also found.
4. Shortly after the appearance of IgG antibodies to gp41, IgG antibodies to p24 (i.e., anti-p24) start to appear. These are referred to as 'core' antibodies.
5. As the level (titre) of anti-p24 rises, the level of p24 antigen decreases to levels which are no longer detectable.
6. Shortly after this, IgM antibody titres also decrease and disappear.
7. Many years will now go by and both IgG antibodies to p24 and gp41 will be detectable.
8. Eventually, IgG core antibodies (i.e., anti-p24) will start to decrease and p24 antigen will re-appear. **It is thought that this serological event is associated with progression into clinical illness.**

Types of Serological Tests for HIV

Any serological test used for detecting HIV infection must have a high degree of **sensitivity** (the probability that the test will be positive if the patient is infected) and **specificity** (the probability that the test will be negative if the patient is uninfected). No screening tests for any trait are ever 100 per cent sensitive and specific and therefore, all positive test results are retested by another method for confirmation.

ELISA ('enzyme linked immunosorbent assay') or EIA (enzyme immunoassay) are the most common tests used for screening for markers of HIV infection. There are several different types of ELISA/EIA tests on the market but they all look for IgG antibodies to the transmembrane glycoprotein (gp41) and the p24 core protein. Special ELISA/EIA tests can also look for IgM antibodies to both gp41 and p24. ELISA/EIA tests are also designed to detect p24 antigen and this test is generally referred to by clients as the **'antigen test'**.

ELISA/EIA tests can be designed to test for markers of both HIV-1 and HIV-2 infection. The sensitivity and specificity of ELISA/EIA tests are generally high but may vary from one laboratory to another. Therefore, a single positive ELISA/EIA result is not presumptive for infection. Diagnosis should be established by repeated positive ELISA/EIA tests and a positive confirmatory test.

The **immunofluorescent assay (IFA)** may also be used to detect HIV antibodies (especially IgM class antibodies) but is more time consuming and requires more expertise than ELISA/EIA tests. It is used more as a research tool than a screening test.

The **Western blot** is the most widely used **confirmatory test**. It uses gel electrophoresis to separate viral antigens and then antibodies to individual viral proteins can be identified. This test is accurate when properly conducted and analysed; however, it is difficult to perform and interpret. **Third generation ELISA/EIA** tests are becoming much more sensitive and specific and may replace Western Blot as a confirmatory tests.

The **PCR (polymerase chain reaction)** is a gene-amplification technique which measures HIV nucleic acid. It can detect minute amounts of HIV genetic material in infected individuals. It is not used as a general screening test but may be useful in detecting HIV infection in infants and in those rare cases where, despite indications of HIV disease, an individual consistently tests negative by ELISA/EIA.

Viral culture techniques can be used to isolate HIV from peripheral blood mononuclear cells (PBMCs), cell-free plasma, bone marrow cells and cerebrospinal fluid. A positive viral culture reflects a true viremia. HIV can be cultured during primary infection or during symptomatic illness. It becomes more difficult to culture HIV during the long period of asymptomatic infection.

A new range of **'rapid method'** tests have now been developed which offer almost instant results and do not require laboratory equipment to interpret. These include **TESTPACK** (Abbott), **HIVCHECK** (Dupont), **GENIE** (Genetic System) and **AIDS-SUDS** (Murex) (7). These will enable screening in a variety of sites where it is not possible to process standard HIV tests. In the UK, TESTPACK (Abbott) is the most widely used 'rapid method test' and will detect markers of both HIV-1 and HIV-2 infection. Calypte Biomedical have also developed a kit for detecting HIV antibodies in urine. Although there is no doubt that the new 'rapid method' tests will be useful, they present unique issues (e.g. home testing) which need to be addressed. However, they offer for the first time a realistic technique for screening blood transfusions in developing countries.

Guidelines for Counselling and Testing

Counselling and testing individuals who are infected or at risk of acquiring HIV infection is an important component of a comprehensive prevention strategy. The vast majority of persons infected with HIV are unaware of their infection. The primary public health purposes of counselling and testing are to help uninfected individuals initiate and sustain behavioural changes that reduce their risk of becoming infected and to assist infected individuals in avoiding infecting others.

The **benefits to the individual** of being tested if their past behaviour may have exposed them to infection include:-

1. An opportunity for individual counselling and health education. Those who test negative may be reassured by their test result and increase their commitment to avoid becoming infected.
2. If their test is positive, regular monitoring of T4 helper cells (CD4 + lymphocytes) can be initiated and individuals so identified can take advantage of current and developing treatment strategies designed to slow down disease progression. An example of this is the introduction of zidovudine treatment for individuals who are asymptomatically infected with HIV and have T4 counts below 500 mm3 (8).
3. In addition, regular monitoring of health status and T4 counts in infected individuals will indicate when to initiate primary prophylaxis for opportunistic infections.
4. Infected individuals can also be immunized against various illnesses (e.g. pneumococcal, pneumonia, influenza and hepatitis B) while their immune system is still capable of responding to vaccines.
5. For women who are infected, this information may be paramount as they make decisions in relation to having children. In addition, cervical dysplasia is more common in immunosuppressed women and HIV infection may be an indication for more frequent cervical cytology[9].
6. For individuals undergoing medical evaluation or treatment, it may be essential to know their HIV status in order to make informed medical decisions. For example, transplant surgery should not be considered for individuals infected with HIV as the associated immunosuppressant therapy would be contra-indicated. Other drugs or treatment may also be contra-indicated. In addition, regular screening for tuberculosis would be beneficial for individuals who know they are infected as HIV infection is associated with an increased incidence of severe clinical tuberculosis[10].

There are also many **individual disadvantages** of being screened.

1. A negative result may falsely reassure and individuals may not follow safer sexual practices.
2. If the test results become known to anyone other than yourself and those personally involved, you risk losing your job and friends and may have difficulty in obtaining insurance (medical, mortgages, etc.). Unfortunately, discrimination against individuals infected with HIV is rampant, e.g. your right to travel to many foreign countries may be restricted, etc. It may be significant to some individuals (or institutions) that you were tested, regardless of the result (the 'where there's smoke there's fire' theory).
3. A positive test result is a heavy burden to carry and you may have psychological difficulty adjusting to this information.

The decision to be tested can only be an individual decision, based upon perceived benefits and risks.

Hospitals and other health care facilities must ensure that they have trained adequate numbers of health care professionals to implement effective pre- and post-test counselling. This textbook is not about the skills needed to engage in counselling activities but excellent textbooks on this issue are now widely available[11, 12].

It is important for nurses to remember that HIV testing has no logical place in making infection control decisions. A person can test negative and yet be infected with HIV for all the reasons described in Table 14.3.

It is for the above reasons and becasue of the increasing number of individuals in the community who are becoming infected with this virus that **Universal Precautions** (Chapters 8 and 10) have become incorporated into current clinical nursing practice.

Table 14.3 HIV Infection in the Presence of a Negative Test Result

---

1. There is a lag between exposure and seroconversion. Although this may be only a few months, it may extend up to six months (or longer). During this time, a patient will test negative but will be infected and infectious.
2. An individual may be free of HIV infection and test negative. However, he/she may become infected the following day and then become infected and infectious.
3. Some individuals who become infected fail to demonstrate IgG antibodies detected by current screening tests (e.g. ELISA/EIA negative but PCR positive). They would test negative but be infected and infectious.
4. The result may be a 'false negative' yet this patient would also be infected and infectious.
5. The individual may be infected with HIV-2 and unless the screening test was designed to detect antibodies to both HIV-1 and HIV-2, it may miss HIV-2 infection.

Informed Consent

No individual citizen must be tested for markers of HIV infection without their true, informed consent. Informed consent implies that the reason why the test is being recommended is clearly explained to the patient in language he/she can understand. Since HIV testing is rarely an emergency, time and space should be built into the encounter so that the patient can consider the information given. Literature clearly describing the advantages and disadvantages of being tested should be left with the patient and an opportunity should be offered for the patient to consult with a trained counsellor. The results of the test should be equally carefully explained to the patient and if the result is positive, appropriate post-test counselling and support arranged. The waiting period for the test result is often filled with anxiety and individuals frequently need support during this period.

Hospitals and other health care facilities must also ensure that they have created, implemented and monitor policies and procedures to ensure that informed consent is obtained prior to testing and that mechanisms exist to ensure the confidentiality of the test. If health care facilities are participating in **anonymous, prevalence data** testing, specific protocols and policies must be additionally established for this type of unconsented testing. Model policies for **informed consent, confidentiality** and **anonymous prevalence data** testing can be found in Appendix 6. The advocacy skills of the nurse are often critical in the area of serological testing for markers of HIV infection. In the 1990s, the 'age of AIDS,' clearly we should all behave towards each other as if we were all infected. This includes our positions on sexual behaviour, infection control and making moral and ethical decisions. We should not be doing anything to our patients that we would not wish to be done to us or our loved ones.

Summary

Although impressive advances are being made in the treatment of opportunistic diseases associated with HIV infection, scientists have not yet developed drugs that will eliminate the virus from the body or restore the ability of the immune system to defend the body against repeated assaults by these pathogens. Until this has been achieved, AIDS will continue to be a fatal disease. Immense international effort is being directed towards the development of a vaccine against HIV but it remains elusive.

There seems little doubt that the escape of HIV from the animal kingdom into the human population represents an uniquely sinister threat to the human race. The advent of AIDS may turn out to be the most significant event of our lifetime.

References

1. Fischl, M.A. (1990). Treatment of HIV Infection, in *The Medical Management of AIDS*, 2nd ed., edited by Sande, M.A. and Volberding, P.A., p. 105, W.B. Saunders Co., London
2. Uandkat, J.D., Collier, A.C., Crosby, S.C. *et al.* (1990). Pharmacokinetics of oral zidovudine (azidothymidine) in patients with AIDS when administered with and without a high-fat meal, *AIDS*, 4(3):229-232
3. Public Health Service Task Force Recommendations (1990). Anti-Pneumocystis Prophylaxis for Patients Infected with Human Immunodeficiency Virus, in *AIDS Patient Care* (April), 4(2):5-14
4. Klein, R.S. (1988). Prophylaxis of opportunistic infections in individuals infected with HIV, *AIDS*, 3(Supplement 1):S161-173
5. *ibid.*
6. Centers for Disease Control (1989). Recommendations of the Immunization Practices Advisory Committee. Pneumococcal polysaccharide vaccine, *MMWR* 38:64-76
7. Kelly, E.B. (1990). The Search for a Rapid HIV Test, *AIDS Patient Care* (February) 4(1):25-28
8. Friedland, G.H. (1990). Early Treatment for HIV - The Time Has Come, *The New England Journal of Medicine*, (April 5) 322(14):1000-1002
9. Bradbeer, C. (1990). Human immunodeficiency virus and its relationship to women, *International Journal of STD and AIDS* (July), 1(4):223-238
10. Centers for Disease Control (1987). Public Health Service Guidelines for Counseling and Antibody Testing to Prevent HIV Infection and AIDS, *MMWR* (August 14), 36(31):511-515
11. Green, J. and McCreaner, A. (1989). *Counselling in HIV Infection and AIDS*, Blackwell Scientific Publications, London
12. Miller, R. and Bor, R. (1988). *AIDS - A Guide to Clinical Counselling*, Science Press, London.

Recommended Reading

The Medical Management of AIDS, 2nd. ed. (1990). Edited by Merle A. Sande and Paul A. Volberding, W.B. Saunders Company, USA

Counselling in HIV Infection and AIDS (1989). John Green and Alana McCreaner, Blackwell Scientific Publications, London

AIDS - A Guide to Clinical Counselling (1988). Riva Miller and Robert Bor, Science Press, London

Appendices

Appendix 1: Revision of the CDC surveillance case definition for acquired immunodeficiency syndrome
(see Chapter 5)

A report by Council of State and Territorial Epidemiologists; AIDS Program, Center for Infectious Diseases, CDC. Reproduced from the Centers for Disease Control Morbidity and Mortality Weekly Report Supplement Vol. 36, No. 1S, August 14, 1987

Introduction

The following revised case definition for surveillance of acquired immunodeficiency syndrome (AIDS) was developed by CDC in collaboration with public health and clinical specialists. The Council of State and Territorial Epidemiologists (CSTE) has officially recommended adoption of the revised definition for national reporting of AIDS. The objectives of the revision are (a) to track more effectively the severe disabling morbidity associated with infection with human immunodeficiency virus (HIV) (including HIV-1 and HIV-2); (b) to simplify reporting of AIDS cases; (c) to increase the sensitivity and specificity of the definition through greater diagnostic application of laboratory evidence for HIV infection; and (d) to be consistent with current diagnostic practice, which in some cases includes presumptive, i.e., without confirmatory laboratory evidence, diagnosis of AIDS-indicative diseases (e.g., *Pneumocystis carinii* pneumonia, Kaposi's sarcoma).

The definition is organized into three sections that depend on the status of laboratory evidence of HIV infection (e.g., HIV antibody) (Fig. A.1). The major proposed changes apply to patients with laboratory evidence for HIV infection: (a) inclusion of HIV encephalopathy, HIV wasting syndrome, and a broader range of specific AIDS-indicative diseases (Section II.A); (b) inclusion of AIDS patients whose indicator diseases are diagnosed presumptively (Section II.B); and (c) elimination of exclusions due to other causes of immunodeficiency (Section I.A).

Application of the definition for children differs from that for adults in two ways. First, multiple or recurrent serious bacterial infections and lymphoid interstitial pneumonia/pulmonary lymphoid hyperplasia are accepted as indicative of AIDS among children but not among adults. Second, for children < 15 months of age whose mothers are thought to have had HIV infection during the child's perinatal period, the laboratory criteria for HIV infection are more stringent, since the presence of HIV antibody in the child is, by itself, insufficient evidence for HIV infection because of the persistence of passively acquired maternal antibodies < 15 months after birth.

The new definition is effective immediately. State and local health departments are requested to apply the new definition henceforth to patients reported to them. The initiation of the actual reporting of cases that meet the new definition is targeted for September 1, 1987, when modified computer software and report forms should be in place to accommodate the changes. CSTE has recommended retrospective application of the revised definition to patients already reported to health departments. The new definition follows:

1987 revision of case definition for AIDS for surveillance purposes

For national reporting, a case of AIDS is defined as an illness characterized by one or more of the following 'indicator' diseases, depending on the status of laboratory evidence of HIV infection, as shown below.

I. Without laboratory evidence regarding HIV infection
If laboratory tests for HIV were not performed or gave inconclusion results (see Appendix I) and the patient had no other cause of immunodeficiency listed in Section I.A below, then any disease listed in Section I.B indicates AIDS if it was diagnosed by a definitive method (see Appendix II).

   A. *Causes of immunodeficiency that disqualify diseases as indicators of AIDS in the absence of laboratory evidence for HIV infection*

      1. high-dose or long-term systemic corticosteroid therapy or other immunosuppressive/cytotoxic therapy $\leqslant$ 3 months before the onset of the indicator disease

      2. any of the following diseases diagnosed $\leqslant$ 3 months after diagnosis of the indicator disease: Hodgkin's disease, non-Hodgkin's lymphoma (other than primary brain lymphoma), lymphocytic leukaemia, multiple myeloma, any other cancer of lymphoreticular or histiocytic tissue, or angioimmunoblastic lymphadenopathy

      3. a genetic (congenital) immunodeficiency syndrome or an acquired immunodeficiency syndrome atypical of HIV infection, such as one involving hypogammaglobulinemia

   B. *Indicator diseases diagnosed definitively* (see Appendix II)

      1. candidiasis of the oesophagus, trachea, bronchi, or lungs

      2. cryptococcosis, extrapulmonary

      3. cryptosporidiosis with diarrhoea persisting $>$ 1 month

      4. cytomegalovirus disease of an organ other than liver, spleen, or lymph nodes in a patient $>$ 1 month of age

      5. herpes simplex virus infection causing a mucocutaneous ulcer that persists longer than 1 month; or bronchitis, pneumonitis, or oesophagitis for any duration affecting a patient $>$ 1 month of age

      6. Kaposi's sarcoma affecting a patient $<$ 60 years of age

      7. lymphoma of the brain (primary) affecting a patient $<$ 60 years of age

      8. lymphoid interstitial pneumonia and/or pulmonary lymphoid hyperplasia (LIP/PLH complex) affecting a child $<$ 13 years of age

      9. *Mycobacterium avium* complex or *M. kansasii* disease, disseminated (at a site other than or in addition to lungs, skin, or cervical or hilar lymph nodes)

    10. *Pneumocystis carinii* pneumonia

    11. progressive multifocal leucoencephalopathy

    12. toxoplasmosis of the brain affecting a patient $>$ 1 month of age

II. With laboratory evidence for HIV infection

Regardless of the presence of other causes of immunodeficiency (I.A.), in the presence of laboratory evidence for HIV infection (see Appendix I), any disease listed above (I.B.) or below (II.A or II.B) indicates a diagnosis of AIDS.

A. *Indicator diseases diagnosed definitively (see Appendix II)*

1. bacterial infections, multiple or recurrent (any combination of at least two within a two-year period), of the following types affecting a child < 13 years of age:
   septicaemia, pneumonia, meningitis, bone or joint infection, or abscess of an internal organ or body cavity (excluding otitis media or superficial skin or mucosal abscesses), caused by *Haemophilus, Streptococcus* (including pneumococcus), or other pyogenic bacteria
2. coccidioidomycosis, disseminated (at a site other than or in addition to lungs or cervical or hilar lymph nodes)
3. HIV encephalopathy (also called 'HIV dementia', 'AIDS dementia', or 'subacute encephalitis due to HIV') (see Appendix II for description)
4. histoplasmosis, disseminated (at a site other than or in addition to lungs or cervical or hilar lymph nodes)
5. isosporiasis with diarrhoea persisting > 1 month
6. Kaposi's sarcoma at any age
7. lymphoma of the brain (primary) at any age
8. other non-Hodgkin's lymphoma of B cell or unknown immunologic phenotype and the following histologic types:
   (a) small non-cleaved lymphoma (either Burkitt or non-Burkitt type) (see Appendix IV for equivalent terms and numeric codes used in the *International Classification of Diseases*, Ninth Revision, Clinical Modification)
   (b) immunoblastic sarcoma (equivalent to any of the following, although not necessarily all in combination: immunoblastic lymphoma, large-cell lymphoma, diffuse histiocytic lymphoma, diffuse undifferentiated lymphoma, or high-grade lymphoma) (see Appendix IV for equivalent terms and numeric codes used in the *International Classification of Diseases*, Ninth Revision, Clinical Modification)
   Note: Lymphomas are not included here if they are of T cell immunologic phenotype or their histologic type is not described or is described as 'lymphocytic', 'lymphoblastic', 'small cleaved', or 'plasmacytoid lymphocytic'
9. any mycobacterial disease caused by mycobacteria other than *M. tuberculosis*, disseminated (at a site other than or in addition to lungs, skin, or cervical or hilar lymph nodes)
10. disease caused by *M. tuberculosis*, extrapulmonary (involving at least one site outside the lungs, regardless of whether there is concurrent pulmonary involvement)
11. *Salmonella* (non-typhoid) septicaemia, recurrent
12. HIV wasting syndrome (emaciation, 'slim disease') (see Appendix II for description)

B. *Indicator diseases diagnosed presumptively (by a method other than those in Appendix II)*
   Note: Given the seriousness of diseases indicative of AIDS, it is generally important to diagnose them definitively, especially when therapy that would be used may have serious side-effects or when definitive diagnosis is needed for eligibility for anti-retroviral therapy. Nonetheless, in some situations, a

patient's condition will not permit the performance of definitive tests. In other situations, accepted clinical practice may be to diagnose presumptively based on the presence of characteristic clinical and laboratory abnormalities. Guidelines for presumptive diagnoses are suggested in Appendix III.

1. candidiasis of the oesophagus
2. cytomegalovirus retinitis with loss of vision
3. Kaposi's sarcoma
4. lymphoid interstitial pneumonia and/or pulmonary lymphoid hyperplasia (LIP/PLH complex) affecting a child < 13 years of age
5. mycobacterial disease (acid-fast bacilli with species not identified by culture), disseminated (involving at least one site other than or in addition to lungs, skin, or cervical or hilar lymph nodes)
6. *Pneumocystis carinii* pneumonia
7. toxoplasmosis of the brain affecting a patient > 1 month of age

III. With laboratory evidence against HIV infection
With laboratory test results negative for HIV infection (see Appendix I), a diagnosis of AIDS for surveillance purposes is ruled out *unless*:

A. all the other causes of immunodeficiency listed above in Section I.A are excluded; *and*
B. the patient has had either:
   1. *Pneumocystis carinii* pneumonia diagnosed by a definitive method (see Appendix II); *or*
   2. (a) any of the other diseases indicative of AIDS listed above in Section I.B diagnosed by a definitive method (see Appendix II), *and*
      (b) a T-helper/inducer (CD4) lymphocyte count < 400/mm^3:

Commentary

The surveillance of severe disease associated with HIV infection remains an essential, though not the only, indicator of the course of the HIV epidemic. The number of AIDS cases and the relative distribution of cases by demographic, geographic, and behavioural risk variables are the oldest indices of the epidemic, which began in 1981 and for which data are available retrospectively back to 1978. The original surveillance case definition, based on then available knowledge, provided useful epidemiologic data on severe HIV disease[1]. To ensure a reasonable predictive value for underlying immunodeficiency caused by what was then an unknown agent, the indicators of AIDS in the old case definition were restricted to particular opportunistic diseases diagnosed by reliable methods in patients without specific known causes of immunodeficiency. After HIV was discovered to be the cause of AIDS, however, and highly sensitive and specific HIV antibody tests became available, the spectrum of manifestations of HIV infection became better defined, and classification systems for HIV infection were developed[2-5]. It became apparent that some progressive, seriously disabling, and even fatal conditions (e.g. encephalopathy, wasting syndrome) affecting a substantial number of HIV infected patients were not subject to epidemiologic surveillance, as they were not included in the AIDS case definition. For reporting purposes, the revision adds to the definition most of those severe non-infectious, non-cancerous HIV-associated conditions that are categorized in CDC clinical classification systems for HIV infection among adults and children[4,5].

Another limitation of the old definition was that AIDS-indicative diseases are diagnosed presumptively (i.e. without confirmation by methods required by the old definition) in 10–15% of patients diagnosed with such diseases; thus, an appreciable proportion of AIDS cases were missed for reporting purposes[6,7]. This proportion may be increasing, which would compromise the old case definition's usefulness as a tool for monitoring trends. The revised case definition permits the reporting of these clinically diagnosed cases as long as there is laboratory evidence of HIV infection.

The effectiveness of the revision will depend on how extensively HIV antibody tests are used. Approximately one third of AIDS patients in the United States have been from New York City and San Francisco, where, since 1985, < 7% have been reported with HIV antibody test results, compared with > 60% in other areas. The impact of the revision on the reported numbers of AIDS cases will also depend on the proportion of AIDS patients in whom indicator diseases are diagnosed presumptively rather than definitively. The use of presumptive diagnostic criteria varies geographically, being more common in certain rural areas and in urban areas with many indigent AIDS patients.

To avoid confusion about what should be reported to health departments, the term 'AIDS' should refer only to conditions meeting the surveillance definition. This definition is intended only to provide consistent statistical data for public health purposes. Clinicians will not rely on this definition alone to diagnose serious disease caused by HIV infection in individual patients because there may be additional information that would lead to a more accurate diagnosis. For example, patients who are not reportable under the definition because they have either a negative HIV antibody test or, in the presence of HIV antibody, an opportunistic disease not listed in the definition as an indicator of AIDS nonetheless may be diagnosed as having serious HIV disease on consideration of other clinical or laboratory characteristics of HIV infection or a history of exposure to HIV.

Conversely, the AIDS surveillance definition may rarely misclassify other patients as having serious HIV disease if they have no HIV antibody test but have an AIDS-indicative disease with a background incidence unrelated to HIV infection, such as cryptococcal meningitis.

The diagnostic criteria accepted by the AIDS surveillance case definition should not be interpreted as the standard of good medical practice. Presumptive diagnoses are accepted in the definition because not to count them would be to ignore substantial morbidity resulting from HIV infection. Likewise, the definition accepts a reactive screening test for HIV antibody without confirmation by a supplemental test because a repeatedly reactive screening test result, in combination with an indicator disease, is highly indicative of true HIV disease. For national surveillance purposes, the tiny proportion of possibly false positive screening tests in persons with AIDS indicative diseases is of little consequence. For the individual patient, however, a correct diagnosis is critically important. The use of supplemental tests is, therefore, strongly endorsed. An increase in the diagnostic use of HIV antibody tests could improve both the quality of medical care and the function of the new case definition, as well as assist in providing counselling to prevent transmission of HIV.

Appendix I

Laboratory evidence for or against HIV infection

1. *For infection:*
   When a patient has disease consistent with AIDS:
   (a) a serum specimen from a patient ⩾ 15 months of age, or from a child < 15 months of age whose mother is not thought to have had HIV infection during

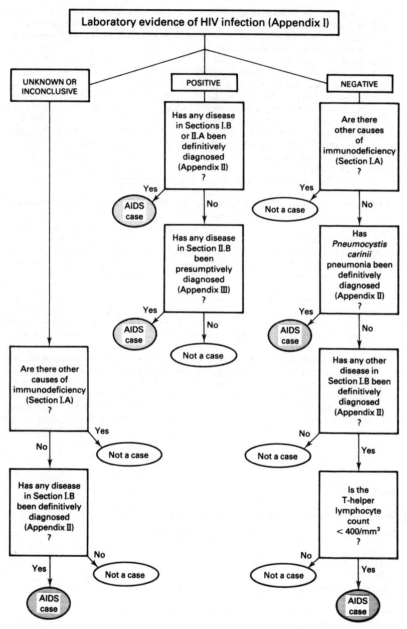

Fig. A.1 Flow diagram for revised CDC case definition of AIDS, September 1 1987

the child's perinatal period, that is repeatedly reactive for HIV antibody by a screening test (e.g. enzyme-linked immunosorbent assay (ELISA), as long as subsequent HIV antibody tests (e.g. Western blot, immunofluorescence assay), if done, are positive; *or*

(b) a serum specimen from a child < 15 months of age, whose mother is thought to have had HIV infection during the child's perinatal period, that is repeatedly reactive for HIV antibody by a screening test (e.g. ELISA), plus increased serum immunoglobulin levels and at least one of the following abnormal immunologic test results: reduced absolute lymphocyte count, depressed CD4 (T-helper) lymphocyte count, or decreased CD4/CD8 (helper:suppressor) ratio, as long as subsequent antibody tests (e.g. Western blot, immunofluorescence assay), if done, are positive; *or*

(c) a positive test for HIV serum antigen; *or*

(d) a positive HIV culture confirmed by both reverse transcriptase detection and a specific HIV antigen test or *in situ* hybridization using a nucleic acid probe; *or*

(e) a positive result on any other highly specific test for HIV (e.g. nucleic acid probe of peripheral blood lymphocytes).

2. *Against infection:*

A nonreactive screening test for serum antibody to HIV (e.g. ELISA) without a reactive or positive result on any other test for HIV infection (e.g. antibody, antigen, culture), if done.

3. *Inconclusive (neither for nor against infection):*

(a) a repeatedly reactive screening test for serum antibody to HIV (e.g. ELISA) followed by a negative or inconclusive supplemental test (e.g. Western blot, immunofluorescence assay) without a positive HIV culture or serum antigen test, if done; *or*

(b) a serum specimen from a child < 15 months of age, whose mother is thought to have had HIV infection during the child's perinatal period, that is repeatedly reactive for HIV antibody by a screening test, even if positive by a supplemental test, without additional evidence for immunodeficiency as described above (in 1(b) and without a positive HIV culture or serum antigen test, if done.

Appendix II

Definitive diagnostic methods for diseases indicative of AIDS

Diseases	**Definitive diagnostic methods**
Cryptosporidiosis	
Cytomegalovirus	
Isosporiasis	
Kaposi's sarcoma	
Lymphoma	
Lymphoid pneumonia or hyperplasia	Microscopy (history or cytology).
Pneumocystis carinii pneumonia	

Appendix II   continued

Definitive diagnostic methods for diseases indicative of AIDS

Diseases	Definitive diagnostic methods
Progressive multifocal leucoencephalopathy Toxoplasmosis Candidiasis	Gross inspection by endoscopy or autopsy or by microscopy (histology or cytology) on a specimen obtained directly from the tissues affected (including scrapings from the mucosal surface), not from a culture.
Coccidioidomycosis Cryptococcosis Herpes simplex virus Histoplasmosis	Microscopy (histology or cytology), culture, or detection of antigen in a specimen obtained directly from the tissues affected or a fluid from those tissues.
Tuberculosis Other mycobacteriosis Salmonellosis Other bacterial infection	Culture.
HIV encephalopathy* (dementia)	Clinical findings of disabling cognitive and/or motor dysfunction interfering with occupation or activities of daily living, or loss of behavioral developmental milestones affecting a child, progressing over weeks to months, in the absence of a concurrent illness or condition other than HIV infection that could explain the findings. Methods to rule out such concurrent illnesses and conditions must include cerebrospinal fluid examination and either brain imaging (computed tomography or magnetic resonance) or autopsy.
HIV wasting syndrome*	findings of profound involuntary weight loss > 10% of baseline body weight plus either chronic diarrhoea (at least two loose stools per day for ≥ 30 days) or chronic weakness and documented fever (for ≥ 30 days, intermittent or constant) in the absence of a concurrent illness or condition other than HIV infection that could explain the findings (e.g. cancer, tuberculosis, cryptosporidiosis, or other specific enteritis).

*For HIV encephalopathy and HIV wasting syndrome, the methods of diagnosis described here are not truly definitive, but are sufficiently rigorous for surveillance purposes.

Suggested guidelines for presumptive diagnosis of diseases indicative of AIDS

Diseases	Presumptive diagnostic criteria
Candidiasis of oesophagus	(a) recent onset of retrosternal pain on swallowing; *and* (b) oral candidiasis diagnosed by the gross appearance of white patches or plaques on an erythematous base or by the microscopic appearance of fungal mycelial filaments in an uncultured specimen scraped from the oral mucosa.
Cytomegalovirus retinitis	A characteristic appearance on serial ophthalmoscopic examinations (e.g. discrete patches of retinal whitening with distinct borders, spreading in a centrifugal manner, following blood vessels, progressing over several months, frequently associated with retinal vasculitis, haemorrhage, and necrosis). Resolution of active disease leaves retinal scarring and atrophy with retinal pigment epithelial mottling.
Mycobacteriosis	Microscopy of a specimen from stool or normally sterile body fluids or tissue from a site other than lungs, skin, or cervical or hilar lymph nodes, showing acid-fast bacilli of a species not identified by culture.
Kaposi's sarcoma	A characteristic gross appearance of an erythematous or violaceous plaque-like lesion on skin or mucous membrane. **(Note:** Presumptive diagnosis of Kaposi's sarcoma should not be made by clinicians who have seen few cases of it.)
Lymphoid interstitial pneumonia	Bilateral reticulonodular interstitial pulmonary infiltrates present on chest X-ray for $\geq$ 2 months with no pathogen identified and no response to antibiotic treatment.
Pneumocystis carinii pneumonia	(a) a history of dyspnoea on exertion or nonproductive cough of recent onset (within the past 3 months); *and* (b) chest X-ray evidence of diffuse bilateral interstitial infiltrates or gallium scan evidence of diffuse bilateral pulmonary disease; *and* (c) arterial blood gas analysis showing an arterial pO_2 of < 70mmHg or a low respiratory diffusing capacity (< 80% of predicted values) or an increase in the alveolar-arterial oxygen tension gradient; *and* (d) no evidence of a bacterial pneumonia.
Toxoplasmosis of the brain	(a) recent onset of a focal neurologic abnormality consistent with intracranial disease or a reduced level of consciousness; *and* (b) brain imaging evidence of a lesion having a mass effect (on computed tomography or nuclear magnetic resonance) or the radiographic appearance of which is enhanced by injection of contrast medium; *and* (c) serum antibody to toxoplasmosis or successful response to therapy for toxoplasmosis.

Appendix IV

Equivalent terms and International Classification of Disease (ICD) codes for AIDS-indicative lymphomas

The following terms and codes describe lymphomas indicative of AIDS in patients with antibody evidence for HIV infection (Section II.A.8 of the AIDS case definition). Many of these terms are obsolete or equivalent to one another.

ICD-9-CM (1978)

Codes   Terms

200.0   **Reticulosarcoma**: lymphoma (malignant): histiocytic (diffuse) reticulum cell sarcoma: pleomorphic cell type or not otherwise specified.

200.2   **Burkitt's tumour or lymphoma**: malignant lymphoma, Burkitt's type.

ICD-O (Oncologic Histologic Types 1976)

Codes   Terms

9600/3   **Malignant lymphoma, undifferentiated cell type**: non-Burkitt's or not otherwise specified.

9601/3   **Malignant lymphoma, stem cell type**: stem cell lymphoma.

9612/3   **Malignant lymphoma, immunoblastic type**: immunoblastic sarcoma, immunoblastic lymphoma, or immunoblastic lymphosarcoma.

9632/3   **Malignant lymphoma, centroblastic type**: diffuse or not otherwise specified, or germinoblastic sarcoma: diffuse or not otherwise specified.

9633/3   **Malignant lymphoma, follicular centre cell, non-cleaved**: diffuse or not otherwise specified.

9640/3   **Reticulosarcoma, not otherwise specified**: malignant lymphoma, histiocytic: diffuse or not otherwise specified reticulum cell sarcoma, not otherwise specified malignant lymphoma, reticulum cell type.

9641/3   **Reticulosarcoma, pleomorphic cell type**: malignant lymphoma, histiocytic, pleomorphic cell type reticulum cell sarcoma, pleomorphic cell type.

9750/3   **Burkitt's lymphoma or Burkitt's tumour**: malignant lymphoma, undifferentiated, Burkitt's type malignant lymphoma, lymphoblastic, Burkitt's type.

References
1. World Health Organization (1986). Acquired immunodeficiency syndrome (AIDS): WHO/CDC case definition for AIDS. *WHO Wkly Epidemiol Rec,* 61:69–72
2. Haverkos H.W., Gottlieb M.S., Killen J.Y. and Edelman R. (1985). Classification of HTLV-III/LAV-related diseases [Letter]. *J Infect Dis*; 152:1095
3. Redfield R.R., Wright D.C. and Tramont E.C. (1986). The Walter Reed staging classification of HTLV-III infection. *N Engl J Med*; 314:131–2
4. Centers for Disease Control (1986). Classification system for human T-lymphotropic virus type III/lymphadenopathy-associated virus infections. *MMWR*, 35:334–9
5. Centers for Disease Control (1987). Classification system for human immunodeficiency virus (HIV) infection in children under 13 years of age. *MMWR*, 36:225–30, 235
6. Hardy A.M., Starcher E.T., Morgan W.M., *et al.* (1987). Review of death certificates to assess completeness of AIDS case reporting. *Pub Hlth Rep*, 102(4):386–91
7. Starcher E.T., Biel J.K., Rivera-Castano R., Day J.M., Hopkins S.G., Miller J.W. (1987). The impact of presumptively diagnosed opportunistic infections and cancers on national reporting of AIDS [Abstract]. Washington, DC : III International Conference on AIDS, June 1–5

Appendix 2: Interim Proposed World Health Organization Clinical Staging System for HIV Infection and Disease

The Global Programme on AIDS of the World Health Organization (WHO) has developed an interim proposed clinical staging system for HIV infection and disease. Following two technical consultations and a validation exercise, a list of clinical markers felt to have prognostic significance was assembled. The list was hierarchically organised into four prognostic categories and a performance scale was incorporated.

An internationally accepted staging system could be used to: improve clinical management of patients; establish reliable prognoses; help in designing and evaluating drug and vaccine trials; and perform studies on pathogenesis and natural history of HIV infection.

The proposed WHO Staging System is primarily based on clinical criteria. Symptoms, signs and diseases should be defined according to medical judgement. Patients, who should be confirmed HIV-antibody positive and 13 years of age or older, are clinically staged on the basis of the presence of the clinical condition, or performance score, belonging to the highest level.

A further refinement of the system would also include, in addition to the "clinical axis", a "laboratory axis". The laboratory axis would subdivide each clinical category into 3 strata (A, B, C), depending on the number of CD4 lymphocytes per mm^3 (>500, $200-500$, <200). If CD4 counts are not available, total lymphocyte counts could be used as an alternative laboratory marker, also in 3 different strata (>2000, $1000-2000$, <1000). Patients would then be classified as 1A, 1B, etc. A suffix should be used to indicate if the laboratory classification is based on CD4(c) or lymphocyte (1) counts (e.g. 1Ac, 2B1). If laboratory values are not available, patients could be classified as 1X, 2X, 3X or 4X, or simply as 1, 2, 3, or 4.

Note: for staging purposes, both definitive and presumptive diagnoses are acceptable. However, if, for a particular disease, the diagnostic criteria stated in the surveillance case definition of AIDS are met, then *the case should be reported on the appropriate form*. In addition, in the UK, clinicians are asked to report deaths in HIV infected persons in whom no AIDS indicator disease was diagnosed either presumptively or definitively.

Clinical stage 1:

1. Asymptomatic.
2. Persistent generalised lymphadenopathy (PGL)

Performance scale 1: asymptomatic, normal activity.

Clinical stage 2:

3. Weight loss, $<10\%$ of body weight.
4. Minor mucocutaneous manifestations (seborrheic dermatitis, prurigo, fungal nail infections, recurrent oral ulcerations, angular cheilitis).
5. Herpes zoster, within the last 5 years.
6. Recurrent upper respiratory tract infections (i.e., bacterial sinusitis).

And/or Performance scale 2: symptomatic, normal activity.

Clinical stage 3:

7. Weight loss, >10% of body weight.
8. Unexplained chronic diarrhoea, >1 month.
9. Unexplained prolonged fever (intermittent or constant), >1 month.
10. Oral candidiasis (thrush).
11. Oral hairy leukoplakia.
12. Plumonary tuberculosis, within the past year.
13. Severe bacterial infections (i.e., pneumonia, pyomyositis).

And/or Performance scale 3: bed-ridden, <50% of the day during the last month.

Clinical stage 4:

14. HIV wasting syndrome, as defined.
15. Pneumocystis carinii pneumonia.
16. Toxoplasmosis of the brain.
17. Cryptosporidiosis with diarrhoea, >1 month.
18. Cryptococcosis, extrapulmonary.
19. Cytomegalovirus (CMV) disease of an organ other than liver, spleen or lymph nodes.
20. Herpes simplex virus (HSV) infection, mucocutaneous >1 month, or visceral any duration.
21. Progressive multifocal leukoencephalopathy (PML).
22. Any disseminated endemic mycosis (i.e., histoplasmosis, coccidioidomycosis).
23. Candidiasis of the oesophagus, trachea, bronchi or lungs.
24. Atypical mycobacteriosis, disseminated.
25. Non-typhoid salmonella septicaemia.
26. Extrapulmonary tuberculosis.
27. Lymphoma.
28. Kaposi's sarcoma (KS).
29. HIV encephalopathy, as defined.

And/or Performance scale 4: bed-ridden, >50% of the day during the last month.

Reference

WHO (1990) WHO Weekly Epidemiological Record (20 July)

Appendix 3: Recommendations for prevention of HIV transmission in health care settings

US Department of Health and Human Services recommendations for prevention of HIV transmission in health care settings. Reproduced from the Centers for Disease Control Morbidity and Mortality Weekly Report Supplement *Vol. 36, No. 2S, August 21, 1987.*

Introduction

Human immunodeficiency virus (HIV), the virus that causes acquired immuno-deficiency syndrome (AIDS), is transmitted through sexual contact and exposure to infected blood or blood components and perinatally from mother to neonate. HIV has been isolated from blood, semen, vaginal secretions, saliva, tears, breast milk, cerebrospinal fluid, amniotic fluid, and urine and is likely to be isolated from other body fluids, secretions, and excretions. However, epidemiologic evidence has implicated only blood, semen, vaginal secretions, and possibly breast milk in transmission.

The increasing prevalence of HIV increases the risk that health care workers will be exposed to blood from patients infected with HIV, especially when blood and body fluid precautions are not followed for all patients. Thus, this document empha-sizes the need for health care workers to consider *all* patients as potentially infected with HIV and/or other blood-borne pathogens and to adhere rigorously to infection control precautions for minimizing the risk of exposure to blood and body fluids of all patients.

The recommendations contained in this document consolidate and update CDC recommendations published earlier for preventing HIV transmission in health care settings: precautions for clinical and laboratory staffs[1] and precautions for health care workers and allied professionals[2]; recommendations for preventing HIV trans-mission in the workplace[3] and during invasive procedures[4]; recommendations for preventing possible transmission of HIV from tears[5]; and recommendations for providing dialysis treatment for HIV infected patients[6]. These recommendations also update portions of the 'Guideline for Isolation Precautions in Hospitals'[7] and re-emphasize some of the recommendations contained in 'Infection Control Practices for Dentistry'[8]. The recommendations contained in this document have been developed for use in health care settings and emphasize the need to treat blood and other body fluids from *all* patients as potentially infective. These same prudent pre-cautions also should be taken in other settings in which persons may be exposed to blood or other body fluids.

Definition of health care workers

Health care workers are defined as persons, including students and trainees, whose activities involve contact with patients or with blood or other body fluids from patients in a health care setting.

Health care workers with AIDS

As of July 10, 1987, total of 1875 (5.8%) of 32 395 adults with AIDS, who had been reported to the CDC national surveillance system and for whom occupational information was available, reported being employed in a health care or clinical labo-ratory setting. In comparison, 6.8 million persons – representing 5.6% of the US labor force – were employed in health services. Of the health care workers with

AIDS, 95% have been reported to exhibit high-risk behaviour; for the remaining 5%, the means of HIV acquisition was undetermined. Health care workers with AIDS were significantly more likely than other workers to have an undetermined risk (5% versus 3%, respectively). For both health care workers and non health care workers with AIDS, the proportion with an undetermined risk has not increased since 1982.

AIDS patients initially reported as not belonging to recognized risk groups are investigated by state and local health departments to determine whether possible risk factors exist. Of all health care workers with AIDS reported to CDC who were initially characterized as not having an identified risk and for whom follow-up information was available, 66% have been reclassified because risk factors were identified or because the patient was found not to meet the surveillance case definition for AIDS. Of the 87 health care workers currently categorized as having no identifiable risk, information is incomplete on 16 (18%) because of death or refusal to be interviewed; 38 (44%) are still being investigated. The remaining 33 (38%) health care workers were interviewed or had other follow-up information available. The occupations of these 33 were as follows: five physicians (15%), three of whom were surgeons; one dentist (3%); three nurses (9%); nine nursing assistants (27%); seven housekeeping or maintenance workers (21%); three clinical laboratory technicians (9%); one therapist (3%); and four others who did not have contact with patients (12%). Although 15 of these 33 health care workers reported parenteral and/or other non-needlestick exposure to blood or body fluids from patients in the 10 years preceding their diagnosis of AIDS, none of these exposures involved a patient with AIDS or known HIV infection.

Risk to health care workers of acquiring HIV in health care settings

Health care workers with documented percutaneous or mucous membrane exposures to blood or body fluids of HIV infected patients have been prospectively evaluated to determine the risk of infection after such exposures. As of June 30, 1987, 883 health care workers have been tested for antibody to HIV in an ongoing surveillance project conducted by CDC[9]. Of these, 708 (80%) had percutaneous exposures to blood, and 175 (20%) had a mucous membrane or an open wound contaminated by blood or body fluid. Of 396 health care workers, each of whom had only a convalescent-phase serum sample obtained and tested ≥ 90 days post-exposure, one – for whom heterosexual transmission could not be ruled out – was seropositive for HIV antibody. For 425 additional health care workers, both acute and convalescent phase serum samples were obtained and tested; none of 74 health care workers with nonpercutaneous exposures seroconverted, and three (0.9%) of 351 with percutaneous exposures seroconverted. None of these three health care workers had other documented risk factors for infection.

Two other prospective studies to assess the risk of nosocomial acquisition of HIV infection for health care workers are ongoing in the United States. As of April 30, 1987, 332 health care workers with a total of 453 needlestick or mucous membrane exposures to the blood or other body fluids of HIV infected patients were tested for HIV antibody at the National Institutes of Health[10]. These exposed workers included 103 with needlestick injuries and 229 with mucous membrane exposures; none had seroconverted. A similar study at the University of California of 129 health care workers with documented needlestick injuries or mucous membrane exposures to blood or other body fluids from patients with HIV infection has not identified any seroconversions[11]. Results of a prospective study in the United Kingdom identified no evidence of transmission among 150 health care workers with parenteral or mucous membrane exposures to blood or other body fluids, secretions, or excretions from patients with HIV infection[12].

In addition to health care workers enrolled in prospective studies, eight persons who provided care to infected patients and denied other risk factors have been reported to have acquired HIV infection. Three of these health care workers had needlestick exposures to blood from infected patients[13-15]. Two were persons who provided nursing care to infected persons; although neither sustained a needlestick, both had extensive contact with blood or other body fluids, and neither observed recommended barrier precautions[16,17]. The other three were health care workers with non-needlestick exposures to blood from infected patients[18]. Although the exact route of transmission for these last three infections is not known, all three persons had direct contact of their skin with blood from infected patients, all had skin lesions that may have been contaminated by blood, and one also had a mucous membrane exposure.

A total of 1231 dentists and hygienists, many of whom practised in areas with many AIDS cases, participated in a study to determine the prevalence of antibody to HIV; one dentist (0.1%) had HIV antibody. Although no exposure to a known HIV infected person could be documented, epidemiologic investigation did not identify any other risk factor for infection. The infected dentist, who also had a history of sustaining needlestick injuries and trauma to his hands, did not routinely wear gloves when providing dental care[19].

Precautions to prevent transmission of HIV

Universal Precautions

Since medical history and examination cannot reliably identify all patients infected with HIV or other blood-borne pathogens, blood and body fluid precautions should be consistently used for *all* patients. This approach, previously recommended by CDC[3,4], and referred to as 'universal blood and body fluid precautions' or 'universal precautions', should be used in the care of *all* patients, especially including those in emergency care settings in which the risk of blood exposure is increased and the infection status of the patient is usually unknown[20].

1. All health care workers should routinely use appropriate barrier precautions to prevent skin and mucous membrane exposure when contact with blood or other body fluids of any patient is anticipated. Gloves should be worn for touching blood and body fluids, mucous membranes, or non-intact skin of all patients, for handling items or surfaces soiled with blood or body fluids, and for performing venepuncture and other vascular access procedures. Gloves should be changed after contact with each patient. Masks and protective eyewear or face shields should be worn during procedures that are likely to generate droplets of blood or other body fluids to prevent exposure of mucous membranes of the mouth, nose, and eyes. Gowns or aprons should be worn during procedures that are likely to generate splashes of blood or other body fluids.
2. Hands and other skin surfaces should be washed immediately and thoroughly if contaminated with blood or other body fluids. Hands should be washed immediately after gloves are removed.
3. All health care workers should take precautions to prevent injuries caused by needles, scalpels, and other sharp instruments or devices during procedures; when cleaning used instruments; during disposal of used needles; and when handling sharp instruments after procedures. To prevent needlestick injuries, needles should not be recapped, purposely bent or broken by hand, removed from disposable syringes, or otherwise manipulated by hand. After they are used, disposable syringes and needles, scalpel blades, and other sharp items should be placed in puncture-resistant containers for disposal; the puncture-resistant containers should be located as close as practical to the use area. Large-bore reusable needles should be placed in a puncture-resistant container for transport to the reprocessing area.

4. Although saliva has not been implicated in HIV transmission, to minimize the need for emergency mouth-to-mouth resuscitation, mouthpieces, resuscitation bags, or other ventilation devices should be available for use in areas in which the need for resuscitation is predictable.
5. Health-care workers who have exudative lesions or weeping dermatitis should refrain from all direct patient care and from handling patient-care equipment until the condition resolves.
6. Pregnant health care workers are not known to be at greater risk of contracting HIV infection than health care workers who are not pregnant; however, if a health care worker develops HIV infection during pregnancy, the infant is at risk of infection resulting from perinatal transmisison. Because of this risk, pregnant health care workers should be especially familiar with and strictly adhere to precautions to minimize the risk of HIV transmission.

Implementation of universal blood and body fluid precautions for *all* patients eliminates the need for use of the isolation category of 'Blood and Body Fluid Precautions' previously recommended by CDC[7] for patients known or suspected to be infected with blood-borne pathogens. Isolation precautions (e.g. enteric, 'AFB'[7]) should be used as necessary if associated conditions, such as infectious diarrhoea or tuberculosis, are diagnosed or suspected.

Precautions for invasive procedures
In this document, an invasive procedure is defined as surgical entry into tissues, cavities, or organs or repair of major traumatic injuries (1) in an operating or delivery room, emergency department, or out-patient setting, including both physicians' and dentists' offices; (2) cardiac catheterization and angiographic procedures; (3) a vaginal or caesarean delivery or other invasive obstetric procedure during which bleeding may occur; or (4) the manipulation, cutting, or removal of any oral or perioral tissues, including tooth structure, during which bleeding occurs or the potential for bleeding exists. The universal blood and body fluid precautions listed above, combined with the precautions listed below, should be the minimum precautions for *all* such invasive procedures.

1. All health care workers who participate in invasive procedures must routinely use appropriate barrier precautions to prevent skin and mucous membrane contact with blood and other body fluids of all patients. Gloves and surgical masks must be worn for all invasive procedures. Protective eyewear or face shields should be worn for procedures that commonly result in the generation of droplets, splashing of blood or other body fluids, or the generation of bone chips. Gowns or aprons made of materials that provide an effective barrier should be worn during invasive procedures that are likely to result in the splashing of blood or other body fluids. All health care workers who perform or assist in vaginal or caesarean deliveries should wear gloves and gowns when handling the placenta or the infant until blood and amniotic fluid have been removed from the infant's skin and should wear gloves during post-delivery care of the umbilical cord.
2. If a glove is torn or a needlestick or other injury occurs, the glove should be removed and a new glove used as promptly as patient safety permits; the needle or instrument involved in the incident should also be removed from the sterile field.

Precautions for dentistry
(General infection control precautions are more specifically addressed in previous recommendations for infection control practices for dentistry[8].)
Blood, saliva, and gingival fluid from *all* dental patients should be considered infective. Special emphasis should be placed on the following precautions for pre-

venting transmission of blood-borne pathogens in dental practice in both institutional and non-institutional settings.

1. In addition to wearing gloves for contact with oral mucous membranes of all patients, all dental workers should wear surgical masks and protective eyewear or chin-length plastic face shields during dental procedures in which splashing or spattering of blood, saliva, or gingival fluids is likely. Rubber dams, high-speed evacuation, and proper patient positioning, when appropriate, should be utilized to minimize generation of droplets and spatter.
2. Handpieces should be sterilized after use with each patient, since blood, saliva, or gingival fluid of patients may be aspirated into the handpiece or waterline. Handpieces that cannot be sterilized should at least be flushed, the outside surface cleaned and wiped with a suitable chemical germicide, and then rinsed. Handpieces should be flushed at the beginning of the day and after use with each patient. Manufacturers' recommendations should be followed for use and maintenance of waterlines and check valves and for flushing of handpieces. The same precautions should be used for ultrasonic scalers and air/water syringes.
3. Blood and saliva should be thoroughly and carefully cleaned from material that has been used in the mouth (e.g. impression materials, bite registration), especially before polishing and grinding intra-oral devices. Contaminated materials, impressions, and intra-oral devices should also be cleaned and disinfected before being handled in the dental laboratory and before they are placed in the patient's mouth. Because of the increasing variety of dental materials used intra-orally, dental workers should consult with manufacturers as to the stability of specific materials when using disinfection procedures.
4. Dental equipment and surfaces that are difficult to disinfect (e.g. light handles or X-ray-unit heads) and that may become contaminated should be wrapped with impervious backed paper, aluminum foil, or clear plastic wrap. The coverings should be removed and discarded, and clean coverings should be put in place after use with each patient.

Precautions for autopsies or morticians' services

In addition to the universal blood and body fluid precautions listed above, the following precautions should be used by persons performing postmortem procedures:

1. All persons performing or assisting in postmortem procedures should wear gloves, masks, protective eyewear, gowns, and waterproof aprons.
2. Instruments and surfaces contaminated during postmortem procedures should be decontaminated with an appropriate chemical germicide.

Precautions for dialysis

Patients with end-stage renal disease who are undergoing maintenance dialysis and who have HIV infection can be dialyzed in hospital-based or free-standing dialysis units using conventional infection-control precautions[21]. Universal blood and body fluid precautions should be used when dialyzing *all* patients.

Strategies for disinfecting the dialysis fluid pathways of the haemodialysis machine are targeted to control bacterial contamination and generally consist of using 500–750 parts per million (ppm) of sodium hypochlorite (household bleach) for 30–40 minutes or 1.5–2.0% formaldehyde overnight. In addition, several chemical germicides formulated to disinfect dialysis machines are commercially available. None of these protocols or procedures need to be changed for dialyzing patients infected with HIV.

Patients infected with HIV can be dialyzed by either haemodialysis or peritoneal dialysis and do not need to be isolated from other patients. The type of dialysis treatment (i.e. haemodialysis or peritoneal dialysis) should be based on the needs of the patient. The dialyzer may be discarded after each use. Alternatively, centres that reuse dialyzers – i.e. a specific single-use dialyzer is issued to a specific patient, removed, cleaned, disinfected, and reused several times on the same patient only – may include HIV infected patients in the dialyzer-reuse programe. An individual dialyzer must never be used on more than one patient.

Precautions for laboratories

(Additional precautions for research and industrial laboratories are addressed elsewhere[22,23].)

Blood and other body fluids from *all* patients should be considered infective. To supplement the universal blood and body fluid precautions listed above, the following precautions are recommended for health care workers in clinical laboratories.

1. All specimens of blood and body fluids should be put in a well-constructed container with a secure lid to prevent leaking during transport. Care should be taken when collecting each specimen to avoid contaminating the outside of the container and of the laboratory form accompanying the specimen.
2. All persons processing blood and body fluid specimens (e.g. removing tops from vacuum tubes) should wear gloves. Masks and protective eyewear should be worn if mucous membrane contact with blood or body fluids is anticipated. Gloves should be changed and hands washed after completion of specimen processing.
3. For routine procedures, such as histologic and pathologic studies or microbiologic culturing, a biological safety cabinet is not necessary. However, biological safety cabinets (Class I or II) should be used whenever procedures are conducted that have a high potential for generating droplets. These include activities such as blending, sonicating, and vigorous mixing.
4. Mechanical pipetting devices should be used for manipulating all liquids in the laboratory. Mouth pipetting must not be done.
5. Use of needles and syringes should be limited to situations in which there is no alternative, and the recommendations for preventing injuries with needles outlined under universal precautions should be followed.
6. Laboratory work surfaces should be decontaminated with an appropriate chemical germicide after a spill of blood or other body fluids and when work activities are completed.
7. Contaminated materials used in laboratory tests should be decontaminated before reprocessing or be placed in bags and disposed of in accordance with institutional policies for disposal of infective waste[24].
8. Scientific equipment that has been contaminated with blood or other body fluids should be decontaminated and cleaned before being repaired in the laboratory or transported to the manufacturer.
9. All persons should wash their hands after completing laboratory activities and should remove protective clothing before leaving the laboratory.

Implementation of universal blood and body-fluid precautions for *all* patients eliminates the need for warning labels on specimens since blood and other body fluids from all patients should be considered infective.

Environmental considerations for HIV transmission

No environmentally mediated mode of HIV transmission has been documented. Nevertheless, the precautions described below should be taken routinely in the care of *all* patients.

Sterilization and Disinfection

Standard sterilization and disinfection procedures for patient care equipment currently recommended for use[25,26] in a variety of health care settings – including hospitals, medical and dental clinics and offices, haemodialysis centers, emergency care facilities, and long-term nursing care facilities – are adequate to sterilize or disinfect instruments, devices, or other items contaminated with blood or other body fluids from persons infected with blood-borne pathogens including HIV[21,23].

Instruments or devices that enter sterile tissue or the vascular system of any patient or through which blood flows should be sterilized before reuse. Devices or items that contact intact mucous membranes should be sterilized or receive high-level disinfection, a procedure that kills vegetative organisms and viruses but not necessarily large numbers of bacterial spores. Chemical germicides that are registered with the US Environmental Protection Agency (EPA) as 'sterilants' may be used either for sterilization or for high-level disinfection depending on contact time.

Contact lenses used in trial fittings should be disinfected after each fitting by using a hydrogen peroxide contact lens disinfecting system or, if compatible, with heat (78°C–80°C [172.4°F–176.0°F]) for 10 minutes.

Medical devices or instruments that require sterilization or disinfection should be thoroughly cleaned before being exposed to the germicide, and the manufacturer's instructions for the use of the germicide should be followed. Further, it is important that the manufacturer's specifications for compatibility of the medical device with chemical germicides be closely followed. Information on specific label claims of commercial germicides can be obtained by writing to the Disinfectants Branch, Office of Pesticides, Environmental Protection Agency, 401 M Street, SW, Washington, D.C. 20460.

Studies have shown that HIV is inactivated rapidly after being exposed to commonly used chemical germicides at concentrations that are much lower than used in practice[27-30]. Embalming fluids are similar to the types of chemical germicides that have been tested and found to completely inactivate HIV. In addition to commercially available chemical germicides, a solution of sodium hypochlorite (household bleach) prepared daily is an inexpensive and effective germicide. Concentrations ranging from approximately 500 ppm (1:100 dilution of household bleach) sodium hypochlorite to 5000 ppm (1:10 dilution of household bleach) are effective depending on the amount of organic material (e.g. blood, mucus) present on the surface to be cleaned and disinfected. Commercially available chemical germicides may be more compatible with certain medical devices that might be corroded by repeated exposure to sodium hypochlorite, especially to the 1:10 dilution.

Survival of HIV in the environment

The most extensive study on the survival of HIV after drying involved greatly concentrated HIV samples, i.e. 10 million tissue-culture infectious doses per millilitre[31]. This concentration is at least 100 000 times greater than that typically found in the blood or serum of patients with HIV infection. HIV was detectable by tissue culture techniques 1–3 days after drying, but the rate of inactivation was rapid. Studies performed at CDC have also shown that drying HIV causes a rapid (within several hours) 1–2 log (90–99%) reduction in HIV concentration. In tissue culture fluid, cell-free HIV could be detected up to 15 days at room temperature, up to 11 days at 37°C (98.6°F), and up to one day if the HIV was cell associated.

When considered in the context of environmental conditions in health care facilities, these results do not require any changes in currently recommended sterilization, disinfection, or housekeeping strategies. When medical devices are contaminated with blood or other body fluids, existing recommendations include the cleaning of these instruments, followed by disinfection or sterilization, depending on the type of medical device. These protocols assume 'worst-case' conditions of extreme virologic and microbiologic contamination, and whether viruses have been inactivated after drying plays no role in formulating these strategies. Consequently, no changes in published procedures for cleaning, disinfecting, or sterilizing need to be made.

Housekeeping

Environmental surfaces such as walls, floors, and other surfaces are not associated with transmission of infections to patients or health care workers. Therefore, extraordinary attempts to disinfect or sterilize these environmental surfaces are not necessary. However, cleaning and removal of soil should be done routinely.

Cleaning schedules and methods vary according to the area of the hospital or institution, type of surface to be cleaned, and the amount and type of soil present. Horizontal surfaces (e.g. bedside tables and hard-surfaced flooring) in patient care areas are usually cleaned on a regular basis, when soiling or spills occur, and when patient is discharged. Cleaning of walls, blinds, and curtains is recommended only if they are visibly soiled. Disinfectant fogging is an unsatisfactory method of decontaminating air and surfaces and is not recommended.

Disinfectant-detergent formulations registered by EPA can be used for cleaning environmental surfaces, but the actual physical removal of microorganisms by scrubbing is probably at least as important as any antimicrobial effect of the cleaning agent used. Therefore, cost, safety, and acceptability by housekeepers can be the main criteria for selecting any such registered agent. The manufacturers' instructions for appropriate use should be followed.

Cleaning and decontaminating spills of blood or other body fluids

Chemical germicides that are approved for use as 'hospital disinfectants' and are tuberculocidal when used at recommended dilutions can be used to decontaminate spills of blood and other body fluids. Strategies for decontaminating spills of blood and other body fluids in a patient care setting are different than for spills of cultures or other materials in clinical, public health, or research laboratories. In patient care areas, visible material should first be removed and then the area should be decontaminated. With large spills of cultured or concentrated infectious agents in the laboratory, the contaminated area should be flooded with a liquid germicide before cleaning, then decontaminated with fresh germicidal chemical. In both settings, gloves should be worn during the cleaning and decontaminating procedures.

Laundry

Although soiled linen has been identified as a source of large numbers of certain pathogenic microorganisms, the risk of actual disease transmission is negligible. Rather than rigid procedures and specifications, hygienic and common-sense storage and processing of clean and soiled linen are recommended[26]. Soiled linen should be handled as little as possible and with minimum agitation to prevent gross microbial contamination of the air and of persons handling the linen. All soiled linen should be bagged at the location where it was used; it should not be sorted or rinsed in patient care areas. Linen soiled with blood or body fluids should be placed and transported in bags that prevent leakage. If hot water is used, linen should be washed with detergent in water at least 71°C (160°F) for 25 minutes. If low-temperature ($\leqslant$70°C (158°F)) laundry cycles are used, chemicals suitable for low-temperature washing at proper use concentration should be used.

Infective waste

There is no epidemiologic evidence to suggest that most hospital waste is any more infective than residential waste. Moreover, there is no epidemiologic evidence that hospital waste has caused disease in the community as a result of improper disposal. Therefore, identifying wastes for which special precautions are indicated is largely a matter of judgement about the relative risk of disease transmission. The most practical approach to the manangement of infective waste is to identify those wastes with the potential for causing infection during handling and disposal and for which some special precautions appear prudent. Hospital wastes for which special precautions appear prudent include microbiology laboratory waste, pathology waste, and blood specimens or blood products. While any item that has had contact with blood, exudates, or secretions may be potentially infective, it is not usually considered practical or necessary to treat all such waste as infective [23,26]. Infective waste, in general, should either be incinerated or should be autoclaved before disposal in a sanitary landfill. Bulk blood, suctioned fluids, excretions, and secretions may be carefully poured down a drain connected to a sanitary sewer. Sanitary sewers may also be used to dispose of other infectious wastes capable of being ground and flushed into the sewer.

Implementation of recommended precautions

Employers of health care workers should ensure that policies exist for:
1. Initial orientation and continuing education and training of all health care workers – including students and trainees – on the epidemiology, modes of transmission, and prevention of HIV and other blood-borne infections and the need for routine use of universal blood and body-fluid precautions for *all* patients.
2. Provision of equipment and supplies necessary to minimize the risk of infection with HIV and other blood-borne pathogens.
3. Monitoring adherence to recommended protective measures. When monitoring reveals a failure to follow recommended precautions, counseling, education, and/or retraining should be provided, and, if necessary, appropriate disciplinary action should be considered.

Professional associations and labour organizations, through continuing education efforts, should emphasize the need for health care workers to follow recommended precautions.

Serologic testing for HIV infection

Background
A person is identified as infected with HIV when a sequence of tests, starting with repeated enzyme immunoassays (EIA) and including a Western blot or similar, more specific assay, are repeatedly reactive. Persons infected with HIV usually develop antibody against the virus within 6–12 weeks after infection.

The sensitivity of the currently licensed EIA tests is at least 99% when they are performed under optimal laboratory conditions on serum specimens from persons infected for $\geq$ 12 weeks. Optimal laboratory conditions include the use of reliable reagents, provision of continuing education of personnel, quality control of procedures, and participation in performance evaluation programs. Given this performance, the probability of a false negative test is remote except during the first several weeks after infection, before detectable antibody is present. The proportion of infected persons with a false negative test attributed to absence of antibody in the early stages of infection is dependent on both the incidence and prevalence of HIV infection in a population (Table 1.)

The specificity of the currently licensed EIA tests is approximately 99% when repeatedly reactive tests are considered. Repeat testing of initially reactive specimens by EIA is required to reduce the likelihood of laboratory error. To increase further the specificity of serologic tests, laboratories must use a supplemental test, most often the Western blot, to validate repeatedly reactive EIA results. Under

Table 1 Estimated annual number of patients infected with HIV not detected by HIV-antibody testing in a hypothetical hospital with 10 000 admissions/year. The estimates are based on the following assumptions: (1) the sensitivity of the screening test is 99% (i.e. 99% of HIV infected persons with antibody will be detected); (2) persons infected with HIV will not develop detectable antibody (sero-convert) until 6 weeks (1.5 months) after infection; (3) new infections occur at an equal rate throughout the year; (4) calculations of the number of HIV infected persons in the patient population are based on the mid-year prevalence, which is the beginning prevalence plus half the annual incidence of infections.

Beginning prevalence of HIV infection	Annual incidence of HIV infection	Approximate number of HIV infected patients	Approximate number of HIV infected patients not detected
5.0%	1.0%	550	17–18
5.0%	0.5%	525	11–12
1.0%	0.2%	110	3–4
1.0%	0.1%	105	2–3
0.1%	0.02%	11	0–1
0.1%	0.01%	11	0–1

optimal laboratory conditions, the sensitivity of the Western blot test is comparable to or greater than that of a repeatedly reactive EIA, and the Western blot is highly specific when strict criteria are used to interpret the test results. The testing sequence of a repeatedly reactive EIA and a positive Western blot test is highly predictive of HIV infection, even in a population with a low prevalence of infection (Table 2). If the Western blot test result is indeterminant, the testing sequence is considered equivocal for HIV infection. When this occurs, the Western blot test should be repeated on the same serum sample, and, if still indeterminant, the testing sequence should be repeated on a sample collected 3–6 months later. Use of other supplemental tests may aid in interpreting of results on samples that are persistently indeterminant by Western blot.

Testing of patients
Previous CDC recommendations have emphasized the value of HIV serologic testing of patients for: (1) management of parenteral or mucous membrane exposures of health care workers, (2) patient diagnosis and management, and (3) counselling and serologic testing to prevent and control HIV transmission in the community. In addition, more recent recommendations have stated that hospitals, in conjunction with state and local health departments, should periodically determine the prevalence of HIV infection among patients from age groups at highest risk of infection[32].

Adherence to universal blood and body fluid precautions recommended for the care of all patients will minimize the risk of transmission of HIV and other blood-borne pathogens from patients to health care workers. The utility of routine HIV serologic testing of patients as an adjunct to universal precautions is unknown. Results of such testing may not be available in emergency or outpatient settings. In addition, some recently infected patients will not have detectable antibody to HIV (Table 1).

Personnel in some hospitals have advocated serologic testing of patients in settings in which exposure of health care workers to large amounts of patients' blood may be anticipated. Specific patients for whom serologic testing has been advocated include those undergoing major operative procedures and those undergoing treatment in critical care units, especially if they have conditions involving uncontrolled bleeding. Decisions regarding the need to establish testing programmes for patients should be made by physicians or individual institutions. In addition, when deemed appropriate, testing of individual patients may be performed on agreement between the patient and the physician providing care.

Table 2 Predictive value of positive HIV antibody tests in hypothetical populations with different prevalences of infection.

	Prevalence of infection	Predictive value of positive test[1]
Repeatedly reactive enzyme immunoassay (EIA)[2]	0.2%	28.41%
	2.0%	80.16%
	20.0%	98.02%
Repeatedly reactive EIA followed by positive Western blot (WB)[3]	0.2%	99.75%
	2.0%	99.97%
	20.0%	99.99%

1 Proportion of persons with positive test results who are actually infected with HIV.
2 Assumes EIA sensitivity of 99.0% and specificity of 99.5%.
3 Assumes WB sensitivity of 99.0% and specificity of 99.9%.

In addition to the universal precautions recommended for all patients, certain additional precautions for the care of HIV infected patients undergoing major surgical operations have been proposed by personnel in some hospitals. For example, surgical procedures on an HIV infected patient might be altered so that hand-to-hand passing of sharp instruments would be eliminated; stapling instruments rather than hand-suturing equipment might be used to perform tissue approximation; electrocautery devices rather than scalpels might be used as cutting instruments; and, even though uncomfortable, gowns that totally prevent seepage of blood onto the skin of members of the operative team might be worn. While such modifications might further minimize the risk of HIV infection for members of the operative team, some of these techniques could result in prolongation of operative time and could potentially have an adverse effect on the patient.

Testing programmes, if developed, should include the following principles:
- Obtaining consent for testing.
- Informing patients of test results, and providing counselling for seropositive patients by properly trained persons.
- Assuring that confidentiality safeguards are in place to limit knowledge of test results to those directly involved in the care of infected patients or as required by law.
- Assuring that identification of infected patients will not result in denial of needed care or provision of suboptimal care.
- Evaluating prospectively (1) the efficacy of the programme in reducing the incidence of parenteral, mucous membrane, or significant cutaneous

exposures of health care workers to the blood or other body fluids of HIV infected patients and (2) the effect of modified procedures on patients.

Testing of health care workers

Although transmission of HIV from infected health care workers to patients has not been reported, transmission during invasive procedures remains a possibility. Transmission of hepatitis B virus (HBV) – a blood-borne agent with a considerably greater potential for nosocomial spread – from health care workers to patients has been documented. Such transmission has occurred in situations (e.g. oral and gynaecologic surgery) in which health care workers, when tested, had very high concentrations of HBV in their blood (at least 100 million infectious virus particles per millilitre, a concentration much higher than occurs with HIV infection), and the health care workers sustained a puncture wound while performing invasive procedures or had exudative or weeping lesions or microlacerations that allowed virus to contaminate instruments or open wounds of patients[33,34].

The hepatitis B experience indicates that only those health care workers who perform certain types of invasive procedures have transmitted HBV to patients. Adherence to recommendations in this document will minimize the risk of transmission of HIV and other blood-borne pathogens from health care workers to patients during invasive procedures. Since transmission of HIV from infected health care workers performing invasive procedures to their patients has not been reported and would be expected to occur only very rarely, if at all, the utility of routine testing of such health care workers to prevent transmission of HIV cannot be assessed. If consideration is given to developing a serologic testing programme for health care workers who perform invasive procedures, the frequency of testing, as well as the issues of consent, confidentially, and consequences of test results – as previously outlined for testing programmes for patients – must be addressed.

Management of infected health care workers

Health-care workers with impaired immune systems resulting from HIV infection or other causes are at increased risk of acquiring or experiencing serious complications of infectious disease. Of particular concern is the risk of severe infection following exposure to patients with infectious diseases that are easily transmitted if appropriate precautions are not taken (e.g. measles, varicella). Any health care worker with an impaired immune system should be counselled about the potential risk associated with taking care of patients with any transmissible infection and should continue to follow existing recommendations for infection control to minimize risk of exposure to other infectious agents [7,35]. Recommendations of the Immunization Practices Advisory Committee (ACIP) and institutional policies concerning requirements for vaccinating health care workers with live virus vaccines (e.g. measles, rubella) should also be considered.

The question of whether workers infected with HIV – especially those who perform invasive procedures – can adequately and safely be allowed to perform patient care duties or whether their work assignments should be changed must be determined on an individual basis. These decisions should be made by the health care worker's personal physician(s) in conjunction with the medical directors and personnel health service staff of the employing institution or hospital.

Management of exposures

If a health care worker has a parenteral (e.g. needlestick or cut) or mucous membrane (e.g. splash to the eye or mouth) exposure to blood or other body fluids or has a cutaneous exposure involving large amounts of blood or prolonged contact with blood – especially when the exposed skin is chapped, abraded, or afflicted with dermatitis – the source patient should be informed of the incident and tested for serologic evidence of HIV infection after consent is obtained. Policies should be developed for testing source patients in situations in which consent cannot be obtained (e.g. an unconscious patient).

If the source patient has AIDS, is positive for HIV antibody, or refuses the test, the health care worker should be counselled regarding the risk of infection and evaluated clinically and serologically for evidence of HIV infection as soon as possible after the exposure. The health care worker should be advised to report and seek medical evaluation for any acute febrile illness that occurs within 12 weeks after the exposure. Such an illness – particularly one characterized by fever, rash, or lympha- denopathy – may be indicative of recent HIV infection. Seronegative health care workers should be retested 6 weeks post-exposure and on a periodic basis thereafter (e.g. 12 weeks and 6 months after exposure) to determine whether transmission has occured. During this follow-up period – especially the first 6–12 weeks after exposure, when most infected persons are expected to seroconvert – exposed health care workers should follow US Public Health Service (PHS) recommendations for preventing transmission of HIV [36,37].

No further follow-up of a health care worker exposed to infection as described above is necessary if the source patient is seronegative unless the source patient is at high risk of HIV infection. In the latter case, a subsequent specimen (e.g. 12 weeks following exposure) may be obtained from the health care worker for antibody testing. If the source patient cannot be identified, decisions regarding appropriate follow-up should be individualized. Serologic testing should be available to all health care workers who are concerned that they may have been infected with HIV.

If a patient has a parenteral or mucous membrane exposure to blood or other body fluid of a health care worker, the patient should be informed of the incident, and the same procedure outlined above for management of exposures should be followed for both the source health care worker and the exposed patient.

References

1. CDC (1982). Acquired immunodeficiency syndrome (AIDS): Precautions for clinical and laboratory staffs. *MMWR*, 31:577–80
2. CDC (1983). Acquired immunodeficiency syndrome (AIDS): Precautions for health-care workers and allied professionals. *MMWR*, 32:450–1
3. CDC (1985). Recommendations for preventing transmission of infection with human T-lymphotropic virus type III/lymphadenopathy-associated virus in the workplace. *MMWR*, 34:681–6, 691–5
4. CDC (1986). Recommendations for preventing transmission of infection with human T-lymphotropic virus type III/lymphadenopathy-associated virus during invasive procedures. *MMWR*, 35:221–3
5. CDC (1985). Recommendations for preventing possible transmission of human T-lymphotropic virus type III/lymphadenopathy-associated virus from tears. *MMWR*, 34:533–4
6. CDC (1986). Recommendations for providing dialysis treatment to patients infected with human T-lymphotropic virus type III/lymphadenopathy-associated virus infection. *MMWR*, 35:376–8, 383
7. Garner, J.S. and Simmons, B.P. (1983). Guideline for isolation precautions in hospitals. *Infect Control*, (suppl):245–325
8. CDC (1986). Recommended infection control practices for dentistry. *MMWR*, 35:237–42
9. McCray, E. (1986). The Cooperative Needlestick Surveillance Group. Occupational risk of the acquired immunodeficiency syndrome among health care workers. *N Engl J Med*, 314:1127–32
10. Henderson, D.K., Saah, A.J., Zak, B.J., *et al.* (1986). Risk of nosocomial infection with human T-cell lymphotropic virus type III/lymphadenopathy-associated virus in a large

cohort of intensively exposed health care workers. *Ann Intern Med*, 104:644–7
11. Gerberding, J.L., Bryant-LeBlanc, C.E., Nelson, K., *et al.* (1987). Risk of transmitting the human immunodeficiency virus, cytomegalovirus, and hepatitis B virus to health care workers exposed to patients with AIDS and AIDS-related conditions. *J Infect Dis*, 156:1–8
12. McEvoy, M., Porter, K., Mortimer, P., Simmons, N. and Shanson, D. (1987). Prospective study of clinical, laboratory, and ancillary staff with accidental exposures to blood or other body fluids from patients infected with HIV. *Br Med J*, 294:1595–7
13. Anonymous. (1984). Needlestick transmission of HTLV-III from a patient infected in Africa. *Lancet* 2:1376–7
14. Oksenhendler, E., Harzic, M., Le Roux, J.M., Rabian, C., Clauvel, J.P. (1986). HIV infection with seroconversion after a superficial needlestick injury to the finger. *N Engl J Med*, 315:582
15. Neisson-Vernant, C., Arfi, S., Mathez, D., Leibowitch, J. and Monplaisir, N. (1986). Needlestick HIV seroconversion in a nurse. *Lancet*, 2:814
16. Grint, P. and McEvoy, M. (1985). Two associated cases of the acquired immune deficiency syndrome (AIDS). *PHLS Commun Dis Rep*, 42:4
17. CDC (1986). Apparent transmission of human T-lymphotropic virus type III/lymphadenopathy-associated virus from a child to a mother providing health care. *MMWR*, 35:76–9
18. CDC (1987). Update: Human immunodeficiency virus infections in health care workers exposed to blood of infected patients. *MMWR*, 36:285–9
19. Kline, R.S., Phelan, J., Friedland, G.H., *et al.* (1985). Low occupational risk for HIV infection for dental professionals (Abstract), in *Abstracts from the III International Conference on AIDS*, 1–5 June. Washington, DC, 155
20. Baker, J.L., Kelen, G.D., Sivertson, K.T. and Quinn, T.C. (1987). Unsuspected human immunodeficiency virus in critically ill emergency patients. *JAMA*, 257:2609–11
21. Favero, M.S. (1985). Dialysis-associated diseases and their control. In *Hospital infections* Bennet, J.V. and Brachman, P.S. (eds), pp 267–84. Little, Brown and Company, Boston.
22. Richardson, J.H., and Barkley, W.E., (eds). (1984). Biosafety in microbiological and biomedical laboratories, US Department of Health and Human Services, Public Health Service, Washington, DC. HHS publication no. (CDC) 84–8395
23. CDC. (1986). Human T-lymphotropic virus type III/lymphadenopathy-associated virus: Agent summary statement. *MMWR*, 35:540–2, 547–9
24. Environmental Protection Agency, (1986). EPA guide for infectious waste management. Environmental Protection Agency, Washington, DC, US. May (Publication no. EPA/530-SW-86-014).
25. Favero, M.S. (1985). Sterilization, disinfection, and antisepsis in the hospital, in *Manual of clinical microbiology*, 4th ed. American Society for Microbiology, Washington, DC. 129–37
26. Garner, J.S. and Favero, M.S. (1985). Guideline for handwashing and hospital environmental control, Public Health Service, Centers for Disease Control, Atlanta: HHS publication no. 99–1117
27. Spire, B., Montagnier, L., Barré-Sinoussi, F. and Chermann, J.C. (1984). Inactivation of lymphadenopathy associated virus by chemical disinfectants. *Lancet*, 2:899–901
28. Martin, L.S., McDougal, J.S. and Loskoski, S.L. (1985). Disinfection and inactivation of the human T-lymphotropic virus type III/lymphadenopathy-associated virus. *J Infect Dis*, 152:400–3
29. McDougal, J.S., Martin, L.S., Cort, S.P., *et al.* (1985). Thermal inactivation of the acquired immunodeficiency syndrome virus-III/lymphadenopathy-associated virus, with special reference to antithemophilic factor. *J Clin Invest*, 76:875–7
30. Spire, B., Barré-Sinoussi, F., Dormont, D., Montagnier, L. and Chermann, J.C. (1985). Inactivation of lymphadenopathy-associated virus by heat, gamma rays, and ultraviolet light. *Lancet*, 1:188–9
31. Resnik, L., Veren, K., Salahuddin, S.Z., Tondreau, S. and Markham, P.D. (1986). Stability and inactivation of HTLV-III/LAV under clinical and laboratory environments. *JAMA*, 255:1887–91
32. CDC. (1987). Public Health Service (PHS) guidelines for counseling and antibody testing to prevent HIV infection and AIDS. *MMWR*, 3:509–15
33. Kane, M.A. and Lettau, L.A. (1985). Transmission of HBV from dental personnel to patients. *J Am Dent Assoc*, 110:634–6

34. Lettau, L.A., Smith, J.D., Williams, D., *et al.* (1986). Transmission of hepatitis B with resultant restriction of surgical practice. *JAMA*, 255:934–7
35. Williams, W.W. (1983). Guideline for infection control in hospital personnel. *Infect Control*, 4 (suppl):326–49
36. CDC (1983). Prevention of acquired immune deficiency syndrome (AIDS): Report of inter-agency recommendations. *MMWR*, 32:101–3
37. CDC (1985). Provisional Public Health Service inter-agency recommendations for screening donated blood and plasma for antibody to the virus causing acquired immuno-deficiency syndrome. *MMWR*, 34:1–5

Update: Universal precautions for prevention of transmission of human immunodeficiency virus, hepatitis B virus, and other bloodborne pathogens in health-care settings (CDC (1988) *MMWR* 37(24) June

Introduction

The purpose of this report is to clarify and supplement the CDC publication entitled 'Recommendations for Prevention of HIV Transmission in Health-Care Settings' (1) (see p. 203).

In 1983, CDC published a document entitled 'Guideline for Isolation Precautions in Hospitals'[2] that contained a section entitled 'Blood and Body Fluid Precautions.' The recommendations in this section called for blood and body fluid precautions when a patient was known or suspected to be infected with bloodborne pathogens. In August 1987, CDC published a document entitled 'Recommendations for Prevention of HIV Transmission in Health-Care Settings'[1]. In contrast to the 1983 document, the 1987 document recommended that blood and body fluid precautions be consistently used for all patients regardless of their bloodborne infection status. This extension of blood and body fluid precautions to **all** patients is referred to as 'Universal Blood and Body Fluid Precautions' or 'Universal Precautions.' Under universal precautions, blood and certain body fluids of all patients are considered potentially infectious for human immunodeficiency virus (HIV), hepatitis B virus (HBV), and other bloodborne pathogens.

Universal precautions are intended to prevent parenteral, mucous membrane, and nonintact skin exposures of health-care workers to bloodborne pathogens. In addition, immunization with HBV vaccine is recommended as an important adjunct to universal precautions for health-care workers who have exposures to blood[3,4].

Since the recommendations for universal precautions were published in August 1987, CDC and the Food and Drug Administration (FDA) have received requests for clarification of the following issues: 1) body fluids to which universal precautions apply, 2) use of protective barriers, 3) use of gloves for phlebotomy, 4) selection of gloves for use while observing universal precautions, and 5) need for making changes in waste management programs as a result of adopting universal precautions.

Body-fluids to which universal precautions apply

Universal precautions apply to blood and to other body fluids containing visible blood. Occupational transmission of HIV and HBV to health-care workers by blood is documented[4,5]. **Blood is the single most important source of HIV, HBV, and other bloodborne pathogens in the occupational setting. Infection control efforts for HIV, HBV, and other bloodborne pathogens must focus on preventing exposures to blood as well as on delivery of HBV immunization.**

Universal precautions also apply to semen and vaginal secretions. Although both of these fluids have been implicated in the sexual transmission of HIV and HBV, they have not been implicated in occupational transmission from patient to health-care worker. This observation is not unexpected, since exposure to semen in the usual health-care setting is limited, and the routine practice of wearing gloves for performing vaginal examinations protects health-care workers from exposure of potentially infectious vaginal secretions.

Universal precautions also apply to tissues and to the following fluids: cerebro-spinal fluid (CSF), synovial fluid, pleural fluid, peritoneal fluid, pericardial fluid, and amniotic fluid. The risk of transmission of HIV and HBV from these fluids is unknown: epidemiologic studies in the health-care and community setting are currently inadequate to assess the potential risk to health-care workers from occupational exposures to them. However, HIV has been isolated from CSF, synovial, and amniotic fluid[6-8], and HBsAg has been detected in synovial fluid, amniotic fluid, and peritoneal fluid[9-11]. One case of HIV transmission was reported after a percutaneous exposure to bloody pleural fluid obtained by needle aspiration[12]. Whereas aseptic procedures used to obtain these fluids for diagnostic or therapeutic purposes protect health-care workers from skin exposures, they cannot prevent penetrating injuries due to contaminated needles or other sharp instruments.

Body fluids to which universal precautions do not apply

Universal precautions do not apply to feces, nasal secretions, sputum, sweat, tears, urine, and vomitus unless they contain visible blood. The risk of transmission of HIV and HBV from these fluids and materials is extremely low or nonexistent. HIV has been isolated and HBsAg has been demonstrated in some of these fluids; however, epidemiologic studies in the health-care and community setting have not implicated these fluids or materials in the transmission of HIV and HBV infections[13,14]. Some of the above fluids and excretions represent a potential source for nosocomial and community-acquired infections with other pathogens, and recommendations for preventing the transmission of nonbloodborne pathogens have been published[2].

Precautions for other body fluids in special settings

Human breast milk has been implicated in perinatal transmission of HIV, and HBsAg has been found in the milk of mothers infected with HBV[10,13]. However, occupational exposure to human breast milk has not been implicated in the transmission of HIV and HBV infection to health-care workers. Moreover, the health-care worker will not have the same type of intensive exposure to breast milk as the nursing neonate. Whereas universal precautions do not apply to human breast milk, gloves may be worn by health-care workers in situations where exposures to breast milk might be frequent, for example, in breast milk banking.

Saliva of some persons infected with HBV has been shown to contain HBV-DNA at concentrations 1/1,000 to 1/10,000 of that found in the infected person's serum[15]. HBsAg-positive saliva has been shown to be infectious when injected into experimental animals and in human bite exposures[16-18]. However, HBsAg-positive saliva has not been shown to be infectious when applied to oral mucous membranes in experimental primate studies[18] or through contamination of musical instruments or cardiopulmonary resuscitation dummies used by HBV carriers[19,20]. Epidemiologic studies of nonsexual household contacts of HIV-infected patients, including several small series in which HIV transmission failed to occur after bites or after percutaneous inoculation or contamination of cuts and open wounds with saliva from HIV-infected patients, suggest that the potential for salivary transmission of HIV is remote[5,13,14,21,22]. One case report from Germany has suggested the possibility of transmission of HIV in a household setting from an infected child to a sibling through a human bite[23]. The bite did not break the skin or result in bleeding. Since the date of seroconversion to HIV was not known for either child in this case, evidence for the role of saliva in the transmission of virus is unclear[23]. Another case report suggested the possibility of transmission of HIV from husband to wife by contact with saliva during kissing[24]. However, follow-up studies did not confirm HIV infection in the wife[21].

Universal precautions do not apply to saliva. General infection control practices already in existence – including the use of gloves for digital examination of mucous membranes and endotracheal suctioning, and handwashing after exposure to saliva – should further minimize the minute risk, if any, for salivary transmission of HIV and HBV[1,25]. Gloves need not be worn when feeding patients and when wiping saliva from skin.

Special precautions, however, are recommended for dentistry[1]. Occupationally acquired infection with HBV in dental workers has been documented[4], and two possible cases of occupationally acquired HIV infection involving dentists have been reported[5,26]. During dental procedures, contamination of saliva with blood is predictable, trauma to health-care workers' hands is common, and blood spattering may occur. Infection control precautions for dentistry minimize this potential for nonintact skin and mucous membrane contact of dental health-care workers to blood-contaminated saliva of patients. In addition, the use of gloves for oral examinations and treatment in the dental setting may also protect the patient's oral mucous membranes from exposures to blood, which may occur from breaks in the skin of dental workers' hands.

Use of protective barriers

Protective barriers reduce the risk of exposure of the health-care worker's skin or mucous membranes to potentially infective materials. For universal precautions, protective barriers reduce the risk of exposure to blood, body fluids containing visible blood, and other fluids to which universal precautions apply. Examples of protective barriers include gloves, gowns, masks, and protective eyewear. Gloves should reduce the incidence of contamination of hands, but they cannot prevent penetrating injuries due to needles or other sharp instruments. Masks and protective eyewear or face shields should reduce the incidence of contamination of mucous membranes of the mouth, nose, and eyes.

Universal precautions are intended to supplement rather than replace recommendations for routine infection control, such as handwashing and using gloves to prevent gross microbial contamination of hands[27]. Because specifying the types of barriers needed for every possible clinical situation is impractical, some judgment must be exercised.

The risk of nosocomial transmission of HIV, HBV, and other bloodborne pathogens can be minimized if health-care workers use the following general guidelines:

1. Take care to prevent injuries when using needles, scalpels, and other sharp instruments or devices; when handling sharp instruments after procedures; when cleaning used instruments; and when disposing of used needles. Do not recap used needles by hand; do not remove used needles from disposable syringes by hand; and do not bend, break, or otherwise manipulate used needles by hand. Place used disposable syringes and needles, scalpel blades, and other sharp items in puncture-resistant containers for disposal. Locate the puncture-resistant containers as close to the use area as is practical.
2. Use protective barriers to prevent exposure to blood, body fluids containing visible blood, and other fluids to which universal precautions apply. The type of protective barrier(s) should be appropriate for the procedure being performed and the type of exposure anticipated.
3. Immediately and thoroughly wash hands and other skin surfaces that are contaminated with blood, body fluids containing visible blood, or other body fluids to which universal precautions apply.

Glove use for phlebotomy

Gloves should reduce the incidence of blood contamination of hands during phlebotomy (drawing blood samples), but they cannot prevent penetrating injuries caused by needles or other sharp instruments. The likelihood of hand contamination with blood containing HIV, HBV, or other bloodborne pathogens during phlebotomy depends on several factors: 1) the skill and technique of the health-care worker, 2) the frequency with which the health-care worker performs the procedure (other factors being equal, the cumulative risk of blood exposure is higher for a health-care worker who performs more procedures), 3) whether the procedure occurs in a routine or emergency situation (where blood contact may be more likely), and 4) the prevalence of infection with bloodborne pathogens in the patient population. The likelihood of infection after skin exposure to blood containing HIV or HBV will depend on the concentration of virus (viral concentration is much higher for hepatitis B than for HIV), the duration of contact, the presence of skin lesions on the hands of the health-care worker, and – for HBV – the immune status of the health-care worker. Although not accurately quantified, the risk of HIV infection following intact skin contact with infective blood is certainly much less than the 0.5% risk following percutaneous needlestick exposures[5]. In universal precautions, *all* blood is assumed to be potentially infective for bloodborne pathogens, but in certain settings (e.g., volunteer blood-donation centers) the prevalence of infection with some bloodborne pathogens (e.g., HIV, HBV) is known to be very low. Some institutions have relaxed recommendations for using gloves for phlebotomy procedures by skilled phlebotomists in settings where the prevalence of bloodborne pathogens is known to be very low.

Institutions that judge that routine gloving for *all* phlebotomies is not necessary should periodically reevaluate their policy. Gloves should always be available to health-care workers who wish to use them for phlebotomy. In addition, the following general guidelines apply:

1. Use gloves for performing phlebotomy when the health-care worker has cuts, scratches, or other breaks in his/her skin.
2. Use gloves in situations where the health-care worker judges that hand contamination with blood may occur, for example, when performing phlebotomy on an uncooperative patient.
3. Use gloves for performing finger and/or heel sticks on infants and children.
4. Use gloves when persons are receiving training in phlebotomy.

Selection of gloves

The Center for Devices and Radiological Health, FDA, has responsibility for regulating the medical glove industry. Medical gloves include those marketed as sterile surgical or nonsterile examination gloves made of vinyl or latex. General purpose utility ('rubber') gloves are also used in the health-care setting, but they are not regulated by FDA since they are not promoted for medical use. There are no reported differences in barrier effectiveness between intact latex and intact vinyl used to manufacture gloves. Thus, the type of gloves selected should be appropriate for the task being performed.

The following general guidelines are recommended:

1. Use sterile gloves for procedures involving contact with normally sterile areas of the body.
2. Use examination gloves for procedures involving contact with mucous membranes, unless otherwise indicated, and for other patient care or diagnostic procedures that do not require the use of sterile gloves.
3. Change gloves between patient contacts.
4. Do not wash or disinfect surgical or examination gloves for reuse. Washing with surfactants may cause 'wicking,' i.e., the enhanced penetration of liquids through undetected holes in the glove. Disinfecting agents may cause deterioration.

5. Use general-purpose utility gloves (e.g., rubber household gloves) for housekeeping chores involving potential blood contact and for instrument cleaning and decontamination procedures. Utility gloves may be decontaminated and reused but should be discarded if they are peeling, cracked, or discolored, or if they have punctures, tears, or other evidence of deterioration.

Waste management

Universal precautions are not intended to change waste management programs previously recommended by CDC for health-care settings[1]. Policies for defining, collecting, storing, decontaminating, and disposing of infective waste are generally determined by institutions in accordance with state and local regulations. Information regarding waste management regulations in health-care settings may be obtained from state or local health departments or agencies responsible for waste management.

Reported by: Center for Devices and Radiological Health, Food and Drug Administration. Hospital Infections Program, AIDS Program, and Hepatitis Br, Div of Viral Diseases, Center for Infectious Diseases, National Institute for Occupational Safety and Health, CDC.

Editorial Note: Implementation of universal precautions does not eliminate the need for other category- or disease-specific isolation precautions, such as enteric precautions for infectious diarrhea or isolation for pulmonary tuberculosis[1,2]. In addition to universal precautions, detailed precautions have been developed for the following procedures and/or settings in which prolonged or intensive exposures to blood occur: invasive procedures, dentistry, autopsies or morticians' services, dialysis, and the clinical laboratory. These detailed precautions are found in the August 21, 1987, 'Recommendations for Prevention of HIV Transmission in Health-Care Settings'[1]. In addition, specific precautions have been developed for research laboratories[28].

References

1. Centers for Disease Control. Recommendations for prevention of HIV transmission in health-care settings. MMWR 1987;36(suppl no. 2S).
2. Garner JS, Simmons BP. Guideline for isolation precautions in hospitals. Infect Control 1983:4;245–325.
3. Immunization Practices Advisory Committee. Recommendations for protection against viral hepatitis. MMWR 1985;34:313–24,329–35.
4. Department of Labor, Department of Health and Human Services. Joint advisory notice: protection against occupational exposure to hepatitis B virus (HBV) and human immuno-deficiency virus (HIV). Washington, DC:US Department of Labor, US Department of Health and Human Services, 1987.
5. Centers for Disease Control. Update: Acquired immunodeficiency syndrome and human immunodeficiency virus infection among health-care workers. MMWR 1988;37:229–34,239.
6. Hollander H, Levy JA. Neurologic abnormalities and recovery of human immunodeficiency virus from cerebrospinal fluid. Ann Intern Med 1987;106:692–5.
7. Wirthrington RH, Cornes P, Harris JRW, et al. Isolation of human immunodeficiency virus from synovial fluid of a patient with reactive arthritis. Br Med J 1987;294:484.
8. Mundy DC, Schinazi RF, Gerber AR, Nahmias AJ, Randall HW. Human immunodeficiency virus isolated from amniotic fluid. Lancet 1987;2:459–60.
9. Onion DK, Crumpacker CS, Gilliland BC. Arthritis of hepatitis associated with Australia antigen. Ann Intern Med 1971;75:29–33.
10. Lee AKY, Ip HMH, Wong VCW. Mechanisms of maternal-fetal transmission of hepatitis B virus. J infect Dis 1978;138:668–71.

11. Bond WW, Petersen NJ, Gravelle CR, Favero MS, Hepatitis B virus in peritoneal dialysis fluid: A potential hazard. Dialysis and Transplantation 1982:11:592–600.
12. Oskenhendler E, Harzic M, Le Roux J-M, Rabian C, Clauvel JP. HIV infection with seroconversion after a superficial needlestick injury to the finger [Letter]. N Engl J Med 1986;315:582.
13. Lifson AR: Do alternate modes for transmission of human immunodeficiency virus exist? A review. JAMA 1988;259:1353–6.
14. Friedland GH, Saltzman BR, Rogers MF, et al. Lack of transmission of HTLV-III/LAV infection to household contacts of patients with AIDS or AIDS-related complex with oral candidiasis. N Engl J Med 1986;314:344–9.
15. Jenison SA, Lemon SM, Baker LN, Newbold JE. Quantitative analysis of hepatitis B virus DNA in saliva and semen of chronically infected homosexual men. J Infect Dis 1987;156:299–306.
16. Cancio-Bello TP, de Medina M, Shorey J, Valledor MD, Schiff ER. An institutional outbreak of hepatitis B related to a human biting carrier. J Infect Dis 1982;146:652–6.
17. MacQuarrie MB, Forghani B, Wolochow DA. Hepatitis B transmitted by a human bite. JAMA 1974;230:723–4.
18. Scott RM, Snitbhan R, Bancroft WH, Alter HJ, Tingpalapong M. Experimental transmission of hepatitis B virus by semen and saliva. J Insect Dis 1980;142:67–71.
19. Glaser JB, Nadler JP. Hepatitis B virus in a cardiopulmonary resuscitation training course: Risk of transmission from a surface antigen-positive participant. Arch Intern Med 1985;145:1653–5.
20. Osterholm MT, Bravo ER, Crosson JT, et al. Lack of transmission of viral hepatitis type B after oral exposure to HBsAg-positive saliva. Br Med J 1979;2:1263–4.
21. Curran JW, Jaffe HW, Hardy AM, et al. Epidemiology of HIV infection and AIDS in the United States. Science 1988;239:610–6.
22. Jason JM, McDougal JS, Dixon G, et al. HTLV-III/LAV antibody and immune status of household contacts and sexual partners of persons with hemophilia. JAMA 1986;255:212–5.
23. Wahn V, Kramer HH, Voit T, Büster HT, Scrampical B, Scheid A. Horizontal transmission of HIV infection between two siblings [Letter]. Lancet 1986;2:694.
24. Salahuddin SZ, Groopman JE, Markham PD, et al. HTLV-III in symptom-free seronegative persons. Lancet 1984;2:1418–20.
25. Simmons BP, Wong ES. Guideline for prevention of nosocomial pneumonia. Atlanta: US Department of Health and Human Services, Public Health Service, Centers for Disease Control, 1982.
26. Klein RS, Phelan JA, Freeman K, et al. Low occupational risk of human immunodeficiency virus infection among dental professionals. N Engl J Med 1988;318:86–90.
27. Garner JS, Favero MS. Guideline for handwashing and hospital environmental control, 1985. Atlanta: US Department of Health and Human Services, Public Health Service, Centers for Disease Control, 1985; HHS publication no. 99–1117.
28. Centers for Disease Control. 1988 Agent summary statement for human immunodeficiency virus and report on laboratory-acquired infection with human immunodeficiency virus. MMWR 1988;37(supply no. S4:1S–22S).

Appendix 4: Social history form (see Chapter 00)

```
┌─────────────────────────────────────────────────────────────┐
│                      SOCIAL HISTORY                          │
│                                                              │
│ Name _____  Age _____          │
│ Hospital identification number _____  Ward _____ │
│ Date of admission/nursing assessment _____ │
│ Address _____│
│ _____ │
│ _____ (Telephone number) _____  │
│ Next of kin and address _____ │
│ _____ │
│ _____ (Telephone number) _____  │
│ General practitioner and address _____ │
│ _____ │
│ _____ (Telephone number) _____  │
│ Admitting consultant _____ │
│ Next of kin informed of admission:    YES/NO                 │
│ Comment _____ │
│ _____ │
│ GP informed of admission:    YES/NO                          │
│ Comment _____ │
│ _____ │
│ Reason for admission _____ │
│ _____ │
└─────────────────────────────────────────────────────────────┘
```

Accommodation

Own   Rented   Private   Council   Sheltered

House   Flat   Room   Which floor? _____

Stairs _____

Toilet (which floor?) _____

Heating _____ Central heating

Cooking facilities _____

Coin Metres for   Heating   YES/NO   Electricity   YES/NO

Accommodation shared with _____

_____

Pets _____

Pets being looked after by _____

Keys to accommodation with _____

Is accommodation now secure?   YES/NO

If no, what action being taken? _____

Employer and address _____

_____

_____ (Telephone number) _____

Does employer need to be informed of admission?   YES/NO

If yes, who is informing employer? _____

Date employer notified _____

Name/position of individual notified _____

_____

COMMUNITY SERVICES

Service	On admission			On discharge	
	Known	Frequency	Informed of admission	Needed	Arrangement
District Nurse					
Health Visitor					
Home Help					
Community Physiotherapist					
Community Occupational Therapist					
Social Worker					
Meals on Wheels					
Volunteer					
Other (Specify)					
Comments:					

SOCIAL HISTORY/DISCHARGE PLANS

Medications	
Medication being taken on admission	Medication to be taken home on discharge

Medications (patient education)

Date/Time/Name and position of individual instructing patient on discharge medications

Date _____ Time _____ Health professional _____

Assessment of patient education:

Does patient understand how to self-administer medications?	YES/NO
Is patient aware of common side-effects of medication and how to detect signs/symptoms of side-effects and reactions?	YES/NO
Has patient been given *written* instructions on how to self-administer medications, their side-effects and how and when to obtain new supply?	YES/NO
If patient on zidovudine (Retrovir – AZT), has he/she been issued with a timed medication device and instructed on how to use it?	YES/NO
Have all medications/instructions been listed on discharge summary to community nursing services?	YES/NO

Transportation: Indicate below arrangements made for patient's transportation home

Ordered by _____ Date _____
If patient lives alone, who will accompany patient home and see him/her safely in their home?

Requisites for health: State discharge status for the following self-care requisites

The need for adequate respiration:

The need for adequate hydration:

The need for adequate nutrition:

The need for urinary and faecal elimination:

The need to control body temperature:

The need for movement and mobilization:

The need for a safe environment:

The need for personal cleansing and dressing:

The need for expression and communication:

The need for working and playing:

The need for adequate rest and sleep:

The need to maintain psychological equilibrium:

The need to worship according to his/her own faith:

The need to express sexuality:

Has patient education on safer sex been implemented?   YES/NO

Needs associated with dying:

DISCHARGE PLANNING MEETINGS

Notes of Discharge Planning Meetings. Enter summary of Discharge Planning arrangements agreed (date and sign each entry)

Original social history assessment completed by:

_____ Date _____

(Nurse to *print* name)

Signature _____

Final Social History/Discharge Plans completed by:

_____ Date _____

(Nurse responsible for safe discharge of
patient – to *print* name)

Signature _____

NB   A copy of this form is to be sent to Community Nursing Service on
day of discharge and original filed in patient's case notes.

Appendix 5: AIDS educational strategies, as used by the Riverside College of Nursing

Aims

Students will be facilitated to explore and develop their knowledge, skills and attitudes related to the care of patients with HIV-related illnesses to enable them to provide a high standard of individualized nursing care in a safe, caring and compassionate environment.

Learning outcomes

The student should be able to:

1. Utilize a knowledge of the nature and transmission of HIV and HIV-related illnesses when assessing and planning nursing care.
2. Effectively demonstrate a knowledge of the prevention and control of infection when planning and implementing individualized patient care.
3. Show an awareness of the differing lifestyles which may influence the needs of individuals.
4. Explore and recognize their fears, feelings, acceptance and prejudices towards the lifestyles and needs of individuals affected by HIV-related illnesses and develop appropriate coping techniques.
5. Demonstrate empathy, understanding and sensitivity in identifying and meeting the special needs of individuals infected with HIV, their family and friends.
6. Participate in identifying and meeting individuals' health education needs and relate these to patient education and primary prevention.
7. Use the above knowledge, skills and attitudes to provide safe, sensitive individualized nursing care.

A wide variety of teaching styles and methods will be used during the course according to the experience and preference of the teacher and the resources available. The use of workshops, discussion groups, seminars, tutorials, videos and clinical supervision and practice will be included.

Stage of preparation	*Content*
Common Foundation Programme	Identification of human needs.
	Sociology and health to include effects of education, lifestyle and occupation on individual health status.
	The use of an appropriate model of care (nursing construct) to meet the health care deficits of individuals infected with HIV.
	Introduction to interviewing and counselling skills.
	Classification, transmission and destruction of pathogens and its application to the individual's response to infection.

The prevention and control of cross infection to include the principles of Universal Precautions.

Care of the patient with local and/or systemic infections.

Introduction to the care of the terminally ill patient.

Ethical and professional issues in nursing to include the district philosophy in nursing policy, patients' rights, consent, confidentiality, freedom of choice, standards of care and professional responsibility and accountability

Care of the patient with HIV and HIV-related illnesses.

Students will be working in practice settings where there may be patients with AIDS or HIV-related illnesses. Their knowledge, skills and attitudes related to the care of these patients will be explored and appropriate guidance and supervision given by nursing staff.

Students are encouraged to share and discuss their practice experiences. This provides opportunities for problem solving, reassurance and information related to nursing practices and policies.

Branch Programmes

Care of patients with AIDS and HIV-related illnesses is presented in greater detail to include both hospital and community care and related health education. Included may be visits to special clinics and specialist speakers from outside support agencies.

As the students progress through the branch their knowledge, skills and attitudes are further developed with the inclusion of:

- counselling, communication and interviewing skills
- the process of grief and the special needs of terminally ill individuals and their family and friends
- the principles of teaching, learning and evaluation
- the application of nursing research and health education to nursing practice and patient education
- ethico-legal aspects of patient care and their effect on the professional responsibility and accountability of the registered nurse.

Community nursing services

Intended learning outcomes.

All qualified nurses, nursing auxiliaries and health care assistants employed in the Riverside Health Authority primary care service will undertake training to extend their knowledge and skills in reference to caring for patients/clients with HIV related illnesses in the community. Staff will also have the opportunity to explore their attitude towards people with HIV infection.

For all groups of staff to gain an understanding of:

1. The nature and cause of HIV infection.

2. The clinical consequences of infection.
3. The means of HIV transmission.
4. The aspects of confidentiality particular to HIV infection.
5. The systems available for obtaining further information and making referrals.
6. All district policies and procedures relating to HIV infection.
7. Clarification of management/professional clinical issues.
8. The attitudes which are necessary for staff to give confident, compassionate and competent care to people with HIV infection; and the factors which prevent individual members of staff from adopting these appropriate attitudes.
9. The implementation of Universal Infection Control Precautions in primary services.

Different staff groups will require further training

1. *For district nurses.* The necessary training to ensure competence – confidence for the administration of intravenous drugs.
2. *For health visitors.* To obtain a knowledge of:
   (a) the possible effects on the health of a pregnant woman infected with HIV and subsequently as a new mother;
   (b) the possible consequences to the unborn and new infant of a mother/father with HIV infection;
   (c) the district's community HIV policy for children under the age of five, and
     i the safe practices required when visiting any client and child at home and undertaking child health clinics
     ii immunization procedures for a baby who is HIV positive;
   (d) HIV and child sexual abuse;
   (e) monitoring health and development of a child who is HIV positive;
   (f) giving appropriate information about HIV transmission to groups and on a one-to-one basis.
3. *For school nurses.* To obtain knowledge for:
   (a) monitoring the health and development of a child who is HIV positive;
   (b) developing safe clinical practice for all children;
   (d) giving appropriate information about HIV to parents, teachers and school children.
4. *For family planning nurses.* To gain knowledge for:
   (a) health promotion in relation to HIV infection;
   (b) developing skills in discussing safer sexual practices with clients.
   (c) The implementation of Universal Infection Control Precautions in Family Planning Settings.

Learning activities

1. Two day orientation programme designed specifically for community staff.
2. All staff to attend day one.
3. All district nurses to attend day two to receive theoretical education and training on the administration of IV drugs. (Practical experience will be arranged in the community).
4. Specific sessions will be arranged as appropriate to meet the particular needs of other groups of community staff.

Continuing education

Intended learning outcome

All qualified nurses employed in the Riverside Health Authority will have an opportunity to extend their knowledge and skills in reference to caring for patients with HIV-related illnesses and will have space in which to explore their attitudes towards those infected with HIV.

Specific training will include:

1. The nature and cause of AIDS and AIDS-related conditions.
2. The clinical consequences of infection and basic skills needed to care for patients with AIDS and AIDS-related conditions.
3. The means of HIV transmission and the adoption of Universal Infection Control Precautions designed to protect patients and staff.
4. Basic health education skills designed to facilitate primary prevention.
5. Clarification of management/professional/ethical issues and exploration of attitudes which may hinder the deployment of confident, compassionate and competent nursing care.

Learning activities designed to achieve the intended learning outcomes:

1. A series of one-day seminars to be planned and implemented on an authority-wide basis which all qualified nursing personnel will be required to attend. This is to be completed within 12 months.
2. Existing orientation programmes to be extended by one day so that the above one-day programme can be included for all newly joined nursing personnel.
3. More in-depth, sophisticated programmes to be arranged for nursing personnel currently caring for patients, with HIV-related illnesses.
4. Staff support groups to be formed for nursing personnel working with patients with HIV-related illnesses and to meet on a regular basis.
5. Managers to identify key employees who require more extensive training and to arrange for them to attend ENB course number 934 (The Care and Management of Persons with AIDS) in the Riverside College of Nursing. This is to include nurse educationalists.
6. All departments within the College of Nursing to designate at least one teacher who will become an expert resource person for HIV education within their programme or department.
7. The subject of HIV-related illnesses to be comprehensively covered in all ENB post-registration clinical courses, ENB short development courses where clinical updating is appropriate and in all staff development programmes.

Midwifery services

Aims

The necessary education to ensure competence/confidence in counselling women regarding HIV.

To obtain a knowledge of:

1. The possible effects on the health of a pregnant woman with HIV infection and subsequently as a new mother.
2. The possible consequences to the unborn and new infant of a mother/father with HIV infection.

3. The district's community HIV policy for children under the age of five.
4. HIV and sexual abuse.
5. Monitoring health and development of a child who is HIV positive.
6. Giving appropriate information about HIV transmission to groups and on a one-to-one basis.
7. Health promotion in relation to HIV infection.
8. Developing skills in discussing safer sexual practices with women.
9. The legal and ethical considerations involved in serological screening of expectant mothers.
10. Pre- and post-test counselling skills.

For neonatal nurses/midwives

1. The possible consequences to the unborn and new infant of a father/mother with HIV infection.
2. Monitoring the health and development of a child who is HIV positive.
3. Developing safe clinical practice for all infants.
4. Giving appropriate information about HIV to parents.
5. The district's community HIV policy for children who are under the age of five.
6. HIV and sexual abuse.
7. The legal and ethical considerations involved in screening neonates for markers of HIV infection.
8. Pre- and post-test counselling skills.

Appendix 6: The Riverside Health Authority Philosophy for Nursing

The purpose of nursing

To support people during the activities and events of life, from birth to death; using skills, strength and knowledge to enable people to maintain their own balance of health, and assist them in illness and disability towards greater understanding and return to autonomy or, at the end of life, to death.

Philosophy for Nursing

The nature of health and ill health

1. People are deeply rooted in the particular circumstances and events of their lives, and in their own social and economic circumstances, and have differing capacities to deal with life's events.
2. Health is multi-dimensional with interdependent physical, pyschological, social and spiritual aspects. Health and illness are normal states in life.
3. Health is a state of balance between self and the environment. In this instance the environment is taken to mean:-
   (a) The physical requirements for living;
   (b) Relationships between family, friends, and neighbours;
   (c) Relationships within a wider societal role, which reflects a person's perceived value by society.
4. Disability, in the absence of illness or disease, is compatible with being healthy.

People's relationship to health and ill health

1. Adults are autonomous, independent and responsible for their own health. The responsibility for the child's health lies with the parents or parent substitute. However people can be overwhelmed by circumstances, lack sufficient resources or knowledge, skills and strength to take appropriate action. The individual may decide not to take the necessary steps. Social, economic, political and cultural factors may prevent appropriate action.
2. The service needs related to health and illness are not static but will vary over time with social, economic and cultural changes and differing expectations of people.
3. The prevention of ill health is achieved through people coming to know the causes and nature of health and illness and their own capacity to take charge of their own and dependants' health.
4. People have the capacity to heal themselves, but may not have the knowledge to do so or be prepared to accept the responsibility. It is important for every individual to know how they perceive their own health and/or their child's health, illness and role in health care, in order to participate fully.
5. Healing does not necessarily mean the curing or eradication of disease or disability. Healing involves knowing and accepting one's strengths and weaknesses and, within these, leading a happy and fulfilled life.
6. People have rights when well or ill. They should be able to make informed choices and understand the consequences of their decisions. Adults have the right not to consent to treatment.
7. People have the right to privacy and confidentiality.

8. People have the right to receive an explanation of their own or child's condition in language they can understand.
9. Dying is a normal event in life. People should be able to participate in discussions about the management of their care, and to make decisions themselves. For children, the participation of the family is particularly important.

The nursing role in health and ill health

1. Nursing views health as a dynamic relationship between the individual, friends, family and the environment. The individual in health or illness is seen within this context. The professional relationship between nurses and people is one of equality, in which people take responsibility for their own health, and towards which nursing will contribute support which is jointly agreed.
2. The aim of nursing will be to assist people in the identification and fulfilment of their own health needs. This may be achieved by facilitating them to use their own resources, either independently from, or supported by, the specialist knowledge of nursing, or linking into the network of other health care professions.
3. To support people means working with them to agree the care appropriate to their needs. Care means assuming a sense of responsibility, being aware, showing interest, being alert to change, and not necessarily direct physical contact.
4. Nursing is concerned with caring for people who are ill, maintaining the health of those who are not ill, and with preventing ill health. It also seeks, through education, to promote knowledge and develop people's confidence in their own ability to effect their longer term health status.
5. The care given should be sensitive to the patient's own needs for autonomy and responsibility for independence.
6. Nursing care will be offered to anyone who is in need of it, regardless of age, sex, sexual orientation, race, religion, political persuasion or presenting illness. Any person who is accepted by the nursing service is owed a duty of care from which nurses may not withdraw.
7. Care will be assessed, planned, implemented and evaluated using an appropriate model of nursing and a systematic problem solving approach.
8. Planning should take into account the person's current medical condition and treatment as recorded in the patient's notes.
9. It is expected that nursing records will be comprehensive, accurate and written contemporaneously.
10. Nurses should ensure that treatment, its implications and the care required, is fully discussed with the individual, and where appropriate, his or her relatives or friends.
11. Any nurse whose conscience is offended by the way a person's nursing care or medical treatment is managed should make this known to the senior nurse manager.
12. In situations when a person is unable to defend or promote his own health needs the nurse may act as his or her advocate.
13. In meeting people's needs nurses have a responsibility to make the best use of finite resources. However there may be times when available resources will not meet assessed need and in these instances there is a responsibility to inform the senior manager.
14. Each registered nurse, midwife and health visitor is accountable for her or his practice, and in the exercise of professional accountability shall observe the code of conduct of the United Kingdom Central Council for Nursing, Midwifery and Health Visiting (U.K.C.C.).

People's needs

1. The need for support in health and illness can be defined by the person, the parent in the case of children, or nurse, and preferably will be jointly agreed. Where these needs are not agreed, the nurse should recheck the professional evaluation against the person's beliefs and capacity, their wishes and their need for dignity and independence.
2. How the support needed might be achieved should also be jointly agreed. There will be times when the need may be agreed but the support cannot be achieved.
3. The need for support may not necessarily be linked to an individual but could apply to a family, or a community of people.
4. In the situation of health and illness people have different levels of need which usually occur simultaneously, although one may dominate, and the nurse will have to use professional judgement to determine any priority.
5. **Physiological and survival needs.**

   These can be in response to physical, developmental, social, economic, psychological, emotional or spiritual distress.
   5.1. To live
   5.2. To be offered assistance
   5.3. To be given refuge or sanctuary
   5.4. To be comforted
   5.5. To be adequately fed
6. **Safety and security needs.**

   These are related to both physical and emotional safety and security.
   6.1. To be safe
   6.2. Not to be hurt
   6.3. To be guided through health and ill health
   6.4. To feel secure
7. **Belonging and affection needs.**

   These are met by the acknowledgement of the essential human being in every individual, even when the person is perceived as being unattractive, difficult or anti-social.
   7.1. To be accepted
   7.2. To belong
   7.3. For friendship
   7.4. To give and receive love
8. **Self-esteem or respect needs.**

   These needs will always be present, but may increase with the degree of vulnerability which is experienced.
   8.1. To retain own identity as an unique human being
   8.2. To have autonomy
   8.3. To know and to understand
   8.4. To be consulted
   8.5. To be creative

Nurses' needs

1. Nurses have the same basic needs as others. Their need for survival, security, belonging, self-esteem and self-actualization must be met to enable them to meet the illness and health needs of people. Fulfilment of them is a joint responsibility of the individual and the Health Authority.
2. Nurses working within a caring environment which allows them to express their individual needs will be better able to provide optimum care.

3. In order to carry out their supporting role and responsibilities nurses must receive relevant education and training throughout their career. Learning in the clinical areas is aimed at integrating the theory and practice of nursing to enable all levels of registered and student nurses to achieve and maintain the competencies necessary for professional practice. Development of these competencies is the responsibility of the individual nurse. Creating the environment which fosters such professional growth is the joint responsibility of the clinical and educational staff.

4. Maximum use should be made of the wide range of experience within the District to develop and enhance the personal and professional development of nursing staff.

5. The ward sister is responsible for the provision of service to patients, towards which the student nurse usually makes an essential contribution. There is, within this situation, an inherent conflict between service and educational objectives particularly in the event of inadequate resources. It is expected that in the acknowledgement of these differing objectives resolution of problems can be achieved.

6. Where clinical experience is required for students, Nurse Management and the College of Nursing have a joint responsibility to identify the resources required for supervision, teaching and assessment and to monitor that these are adequate. Where resources are inadequate it is expected that nurse management and the College of Nursing will undertake joint action.

Inter-professional collaboration

1. People's needs are often multidisciplinary and health care plans will require input from other professionals. Nursing staff will expect to work, and participate fully, within a multidisciplinary setting.

2. Where the nursing assessment identifies the need for consultation with other health care professionals, the nurse has a responsibility to initiate this and monitor that the changing needs of the person are being met. Assessment of health care needs is best made jointly between the person, the parent/informal carer, the nurse and members of other professions prior to joint agreement on how it will be provided.

3. In a multidisciplinary situation, effective communication is essential to a successful outcome. Nursing, the role of which is continuous and central to the provision of health care, has a particular opportunity to facilitate this.

4. In addition people quickly identify each role and select what is seen to be appropriate knowledge for each. Thus no one worker comes to see the whole picture. It is important that information is shared and this is probably best achieved through agreement on having a key worker or primary nurse.

5. All nurses have specialist knowledge, but the specialist nurse has the opportunity to keep abreast of changes in current practice and to develop a broad range of skills related to that practice. The role is both educational and advisory and offers support to colleagues, other health care professionals, people and families. They are also concerned with the development of resources and liaison between institution and community, health care and social services. Clinical care is given to facilitate learning.

6. The specialist nurse role requires that mutual understanding of, and respect for, others' roles and expertise is established. Where there is dual responsibility for care then entry into that care and withdrawal from it should be negotiated between professionals. This will clarify roles for client and worker and be in accord with a holistic approach to care.

7. Admissions for treatment should be arranged in the best interest of the people

concerned, and should take into account their general and specialist nursing needs. People should be cared for within an environment which has the facilities and specialist skills to meet their particular identified nursing and medical needs.

8. The senior nurse on duty should ensure that nursing, medical and other staff are aware of agreed policies. The nurse can advise the appropriate professional manager if these are not followed.

9. Discharges must be planned in the best interest of people. Nurses have a duty, in liaison with medical, paramedical staff, and relatives/friends, to be satisfied that the conditions to which the person is returning are safe, and to state and document their views.

10. Nurses have a responsibility to ensure that discharge teaching has been carried out and is documented; and that the person and parent/informal carer/family have full understanding of what they have been taught.

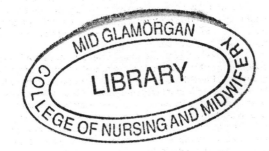

Appendix 7: Policy Statements

A Message from The Chief Nurse Adviser

Dear Colleague

In the United Kingdom, The Riverside Health Authority is at the very epicentere of the current pandemic of HIV Disease. We are currently caring for large numbers of individuals who are unwell as a result of HIV infection and our projections indicate that we will continue to do so for many years to come.

From the beginning of the epidemic, the nursing services within the Riverside Health Authority have endeavoured to create an ethical framework to clarify some of the difficult issues encountered in caring for patients and clients with HIV Disease. Consequently, the Nursing Advisory Committee has created a set of policy statements which describe a model for professional decision making in relation to HIV infection.

This pamphlet describes the principles nurses must consider in relation to:

- Duty of Care
- Confidentiality
- Unlinked Anonymous Testing
- The Employment of Nursing Staff with HIV Infection
- Infection Control
- Informed Consent
- AIDS and cytomegalovirus

These principles are based upon our stated mission of care which is described in the **Philosophy For Nursing** for the Riverside Health Authority (2nd edition, 1990).

The issues which nurses confront in caring for individuals with HIV Disease are not new issues. HIV Disease has merely highlighted the need to re-explore our professional response to these problems. The principles outlined in these Policy Statements equally apply to all the patients/clients of the Authority, regardless of their clinical presentation.

I would urge all nurses and other Health Care Professionals to read these policy statements carefully and ensure that their enactment leads to the continuation of our stated policy that all our patients/clients receive the high quality of care for which the Riverside Health Authority is so justifiably proud.

Chris Beasley   June 1990
Chief Nurse Adviser

Universal Precautions: HIV Disease

The number of individuals in the community who are asymptomatically infected with HIV is *increasing* and it is likely that many patients/clients in hospital or the community, infected with HIV, are unaware of it. Consequently, we would also be unaware of their infection. The current trend is for the prevalence of asymptomatic HIV infection to continue to increase within the community served by the Riverside Health Authority.

It is not the policy of this Health Authority to routinely screen all patients/clients. Serological testing for markers of HIV infection could not reliably detect all those who are infected as a negative test does not necessarily indicate that an individual is not infected with HIV.

Therefore, it is important that all nursing personnel take reasonable precautions against exposure to blood and certain body fluids from ALL patients, in ALL departments, ALL of the time, regardless of what is or is not known regarding their serological status in relation to HIV infection.

Universal Precautions require that nursing personnel wear non-sterile, disposable latex or vinyl gloves whenever exposure to blood or to the body fluids mentioned below is anticipated.

Universal Precautions apply to blood and to other body fluids containing visible blood. Universal Precautions *also* apply to tissues and to cerebrospinal (CSF), synovial, pleural, peritoneal, pericardial and amniotic fluids.

BLOOD IS THE SINGLE MOST IMPORTANT SOURCE OF HIV and other blood-borne pathogens (e.g. HBV) in the occupational setting. The prevention of exposure to *all* blood and to the above *body fluids* is in line with current standards of nursing practice.

All nursing personnel should take precautions to prevent injuries caused by needles, scapels and other sharp instruments. Additional precautions may be appropriate during procedures that are likely to generate aerosol contamination with blood or body fluids.

Universal Precautions are part of the routine infection control advice described in the leaflet **"Universal Infection Control Precautions"** (Nursing Advisory Committee, March 1989). For more detailed advice, nursing personnel should consult the Senior Nurses for Infection Control. *Inappropriate and over-zealous infection control precautions are to be discouraged.*

All nursing service personnel are obligated to comply with current 'Infection Control Policies and Procedures' including this advisory statement. The Nursing Advisory Committee for the Riverside Health Authority wishes this Policy Statement to be discussed with all nursing service personnel within the Authority. All Sisters/Charge Nurses and Nurse Managers must ensure that their nursing staff are familiar with this advice and that 'Universal Precautions' are incorporated into routine nursing practice.

References

Nursing Advisory Committee (1989) **Universal Infection Control Precautions**, Riverside Health Authority, March, London

Department of Health (1990) **Guidance for Clinical Health Care Workers: Protection against infection with HIV and Hepatitis Viruses**, Expert Advisory Group on AIDS (EAGA), January, HMSO, London

CDC (1987) Recommendations for Prevention of HIV Transmission in Health Care Settings, **MMWR** 36(2S) August, USA

CDC (1988) Update: Universal Precautions for Prevention of Human Immunodeficiency Virus, Hepatitis B Virus, and Other Blood-borne Pathogens in Health-Care Settings, **MMWR** 37(24), June, USA

CDC (1989) Guidelines for Preventation of Transmission of Human Immunodeficiency Virus and Hepatitis B virus to Health-Care and Public-Safety Workers, **MMWR** 38(S-6), 23 June, USA

Duty of Care

The philosophy of nursing service within the Riverside Health Authority embraces the concept that skilled nursing care is available to all individuals requiring it, regardless of their race, religion, age, sexual or political orientation or disease presentation.

Nursing personnel do not have the right to decide which patients they will care for and which patients they will not care for. Nursing personnel have a duty of care towards all patients and are professionally obligated to offer appropriate and meaningful care to those requiring it.

All nurses have an individual responsibility to remain clinically up-to-date and to be aware of the policies and procedures for caring for patients with HIV-related illnesses. Refusing to care for any patients within the Riverside Health Authority will lead to disciplinary action by both the Health Authority and the United Kingdom Central Council for Nursing, Midwifery and Health Visiting.

Nurses are reminded that it is both the philosophy and intention of the nursing service in this Health Authority to offer competent, compassionate and non-judgemental care to *all of our patients.*

Confidentiality

All nurses employed by the Riverside Health Authority have both a legal and a profes-sional responsibility to observe **The Code of Professional Conduct for the Nurse** (2nd edition) published by the United Kingdom Central Council for Nursing, Midwifery and Health Visiting. One of the key statements (Clause 9) in this code concerns **Confidentiality**. It reads:-

> "**Each registered nurse, midwife and health visitor is accountable for his or her practice, and, in the exercise of professional accountability shall:**
> **Repect confidential information obtained in the course of professional practice and refrain from disclosing such information without the consent of the patient/client, or a person entitled to act on his/her behalf, except where disclosure is required by law or by the order of a court or is necessary in the public interest.**"

It can be seen from the general description of the Code of Professional Conduct and the particular contents of Clause 9 that **breaches of confidentiality should be regarded as exceptional,** only occurring after careful consideration and discussion with senior nurse managers and other practitioners directly involved in the clinical care of the patient/client.

Clearly it is impractical to obtain the consent of the patient/client every time that health care information needs to be shared with other health professionals, or other staff involved in the health care of that patient/client. Consent in these instances can be implied, provided that it is known and understood by the patients/clients that such information needs to be made available to others involved in the delivery of his/her care. Patients/clients have a right to know the standards of confidentiality maintained by those providing their care, and these standards should be made known by the health professional at the first point of contact.

When an individual practitioner considers that it is necessary to obtain the **explicit consent** of a patient/client before disclosing specific information, it is the responsibility of the practitioner to ensure that the patient/client can make as informed a response as possible as to whether that information can be disclosed or withheld.

It is essential that nurses, midwives and health visitors recognise the fundamental right of their patients or clients to information about them being kept private and secure. This point is sharply reinforced by only brief consideration of the personal, social or legal repercussions which might follow unauthorised disclosure of informa-tion concerning a person's health or illness.

The care of confidential information includes ensuring or helping to ensure that record keeping systems are not such as to make the release of information possible or likely. Neither technology nor management convenience should be allowed to determine principles. Each practitioner has a responsibility to recognise that risks exist, and to satisfy himself or herself in respect of the system for storage and move-ment of records operated in the health care setting in which he or she works and to ensure that it is secure. The concern for the environment of care for which each practitioner is held accountable under the terms of **clause 10** of the Code of

Professional Conduct for the Nurse, Midwife and Health Visitor extends to include this.

The practitioner should act so as to ensure that he/she does not become a channel through which confidential information obtained in the course of professional practice is inadvertently released. The dangerous consequences of careless talk in public places cannot be overstated.

Where access to the records of patients or clients is necessary so that students may be assisted to achieve the necessary knowledge and competence it must be recognised that the same principles of confidentiality stated earlier extend to them and their teachers. The same applies to those engaged in research. It is incumbent on the practitioner(s) responsible for the security of the information contained in these records to ensure that access to it is closely supervised, and occurs within the context of the teacher and student undertaking to respect its confidentiality, and in knowledge of the fact that the teacher has accepted responsibility to ensure that students understand the requirement for confidentiality and the need to observe policies for the handling and storage of records. it is expected that the student or teacher who is active in giving care as a practitioner will apprise the patient of their role, thus enabling the patient who is so capable to control the information flow. Where deemed necessary the recipient of confidential information from a patient/client will advise him/her that the information will be conveyed to the nurse, midwife or health visitor involved in his/her care on a continuing basis.

Confidentiality is a rule with certain exceptions

The needs of the community can, on occasions, take precedence over the individual's rights as, for example, when a Court order demands that a professional confidence be broken.

It is essential that before determining that a particular set of circumstances constitute such an exception, the practitioner is satisfied that the best interests of the patient/client are served thereby or the wider public interest necessitates disclosure.

In all cases where the practitioner deliberately discloses or withholds information in what he/she believes is the public interest, he/she **must be able to justify the decision and must always consult with their senior nurse managers before making this decision.**

If confidential information is deliberately disclosed without the consent of the patient/client, he/she should be informed that this is being done and the recipient of the information should be informed that it is being given to them without the consent of the patient/client.

Summary of the principles on which to base professional judgement in matters of confidentiality

1. That a patient/client has a right to expect that information given in confidence will be used only for the purpose for which it was given and will not be released to others without their consent.
2. That practitioners recognise the fundamental right of their patients/clients to have information about them held in secure and private storage.
3. That, where it is deemed appropriate to share information obtained in the course of professional practice with other health or social work practitioners, the practitioner who obtained the information must ensure before its release that it is being imparted in strict professional confidence and for a specific purpose.
4. That the responsibility to either disclose or withhold confidential information in

the public interest lies with the individual practitioner, that they cannot delegate the decision, and that they cannot be required by a superior to disclose or withhold information against their will.

5. That a practitioner who chooses to breach the basic principle of confidentiality in the belief that it is necessary in the public interest must have considered the matter sufficiently to justify that decision.

6. That deliberate breaches of confidentiality other than with the consent of the patient/client should be exceptional.

References:

Code of Professional Conduct for the Nurse, Midwife and Health Visitor, 2nd ed. (Nov. 1984) United Kingdom Central Council for Nursing, Midwifery and Health Visiting.

Confidentiality – An Elaboration of Clause 9 of the Second Edition of the UKCC's Code of Professional Conduct for the Nurse, Midwife and Health Visitor – A UKCC Advisory Paper (1987) United Kingdom Central Council for Nursing, Midwifery and Health Visiting.

Guidelines on Confidentiality in Nursing (1980) The Royal College of Nursing.

Gillon, R. (1987) **AIDS and Medical Confidentiality**, British Medical Journal (27 June) 294(6588): 1675–77.

Consent for Serological Testing

Nurses must not take blood or collude with other professionals in obtaining blood for serological testing for antibodies to HIV ('anti-HIV') or HIV antigens unless patients have given consent for this procedure.

Consent implies that the reason why the test is desired is carefully explained to the patient/client, the results are made known to the patient/client in counselling sessions and that he/she agrees to this test and understands its significance.

The United Kingdom Central Council for Nursing, Midwifery and Health Visiting have advised nurses that on the specific issue of taking blood for testing **without consent**, the Council advises nurses, midwives and health visitors on its professional register that they expose themselves to the risk of civil action for damages or criminal charges of assault if they personally take the blood specimens, and of aiding and abetting such an assault if they knowingly collude with a doctor in obtaining such specimens.

Additionally, those actions (like that of being party to any statements aimed at leading patients to believe that blood specimens taken for HIV testing were for some other purpose) expose nurses, midwives and health visitors to the possibility of complaints to their registration body, alleging misconduct, which would put their registration status and right to practise at risk.

If any nurse employed by The Riverside Health Authority is **unsure** as to whether or not patients/clients are being asked for their consent to serological testing for anti-HIV or HIV antigens, they should discuss this initially with the medical staff who have ordered the investigation and if necessary, consult their senior nurse manager.

In respect of other aspects of the treatment and care of patients known to be or suspected of being infected with HIV, the UKCC has reminded those on its register that the first two clauses in its Code of Professional Conduct state:

"Each registered nurse, midwife and health visitor is **accountable of his or her practice** and, in the exercise of professional accountability shall:
  Act always in such a way as to promote and safeguard the well-being and interest of patients/clients;
  and

Ensure that **no action or omission** on their past, within their sphere of influence, **is detrimental** to the condition or safety of their patients/clients.

Unlinked anonymous testing for the prevalance of the human immunodeficiency virus (HIV)

Surveillance testing for the prevalence of the Human Immunodeficiency Virus (HIV-1) will be carried out in several Health Authorities in the United Kingdom, including the Riverside Health Authority. These surveys, which have been designed by the Medical Research Council at the request of the Health Departments, are intended to accurately determine the prevalence of HIV infection in the general population. Present data, collected from people who come forward voluntarily for HIV tests, do not give a complete picture and the actual number of infected individuals is thought to be higher than the number reported. More accurate data will assist the Health Departments in planning services for people with HIV Disease and action to prevent further spread of HIV.

Unlinked Anonymous HIV surveys will use blood that has been taken from patients for specified diagnostic or treatment purposes (e.g. Complete Blood Counts, etc.). After the specified test has been carried out, the residual specimen will be stripped of any identifying factors (i.e., anonymised) and may then be tested for markers of HIV infection. It is 'unlinked' in the respect that the results of the tests will not be able to be associated with an identified individual. A further safeguard to anonymity is that the person who tests the batches of samples will not be the same as the person who anonymises them.

The Nursing Advisory Committee supports unlinked anonymous prevalence data testing for HIV infection **only if the below listed requirements are met:-**

[1] A specific protocol for each test group (e.g. pregnant women, newborn infants, etc.) must have been approved by the local ethical committee of the health authority from which the blood specimens are to be obtained prior to the commencement of any unlinked anonymous test programme.

[2] No extra blood will be taken for HIV prevalence data testing; the amount of blood taken on any occasion should be only that which would normally be taken for the specific tests ordered by the patient's medical practitioner.

[3] It is made known to those whose blood may be used (and in the case of children, their parents/guardians) that this surveillance programme is taking place, to explain it and to assure them of the absolute anonymity of the samples used. This is to be done by posters in clinics and units of service selected for prevalence data testing and by giving all patients a copy of the Department of Health Leaflet (AHT1, December 1989) entitled **"If You Are Having A Blood Test"**. Posters and leaflets must be available in the full range of relevant languages appropriate to the known patient/client population.

[4] All nursing personnel assigned to clinics and units of service where prevalence data testing will take place will have received a copy of this **policy statement** and a copy of the Department of Health Leaflet (AHT4, December 1989) **"Unlinked Anonymous HIV Surveys – Guidance For Health Service Staff"**. Nursing Personnel must also be aware of Guidelines from the Professional Conduct and Registration Division of the United Kingdom Central Council for Nursing, Midwifery and Health Visiting (PC/89/01, October 1989 **"Anonymous Testing For the Prevalence of the Human Immunodeficiency Virus – HIV)**. In addition, all nursing personnel will have had an opportunity of discussing the procedures for unlinked anonymous testing with their nurse manager.

[5] All registered nurses, midwives and health visitors assigened to units of service

from which samples are being obtained for this prevalence testing programme must be made aware of that fact in order

5.1 that they may answer honestly any questions put to them by patients and clients about the full range of purposes for which blood samples will or may be tested, and

5.2 they may consider how best to act to protect the interests of any patients or clients whose transient or permanent condition results in an inability to consider and/or understand the available information literature.

[6] All posters, leaflets and verbal advice given to patients/cleints will clearly inform them of *their right to opt out of this screening programme*.

[7] That any patient or client who objects to participation in the test programme must have his or her wishes respected fully and should not:

7.1 be discriminated against in any way

7.2 be identified as being a higher risk than those who have not objected and

7.3 have required treatment withheld or suffer any other detriment.

[8] That there must be no possible detriment to those whose blood is or is not screened as part of the unlinked anonymous testing programme.

[9] If the patient or client wishes, a personal or named test for markers of HIV infection will be arranged, with the required pre and post test counselling.

Confidentiality

The sample from the patient or client will be anonymised. Consequently, as no sample can be linked to any individual client or patient, there is no problem about keeping the result confidential as nobody will know whose result it is.

Consent

The leaflet given to each patient or client (Department of Health AHT1) makes it clear that a patient or client can refuse to take part in the testing programme. *Such a refusal must be respected*. The request form must clearly state that the blood sample is not to be used for anonymous HIV testing. Apart from this, no record must be made.

UKCC (Professional Conduct and Registration Division) PC/89/01 *Anonymous Testing For The Prevalence of the Human Immuno-Deficiency Virus (HIV)* October 1989.

Heptonstall, J. & Gill, O.N. (1989). The Legal and Ethical Basis for Unlinked Anonymous HIV Testing, *CDR* (1 December) **89**/48:3–6.

The Employment of Nursing Personnel Infected with HIV

1. In May, 1988, The Riverside Health Authority issued guidelines for managers in relation to health authority personnel infected with HIV. Guidelines have also been issued by the Department of Health, the World Health Organisation, the Department of Employment and the Health and Safety Executive and the United Kingdom Central Council for Nursing, Midwifery and Health Visiting.

2. The following guidelines are compatible with the above and seek to clarify the employment issues for nursing personnel infected with HIV.

3. Protection of the human rights and dignity of HIV-infected persons, including persons with AIDS, is essential for prevention and control of HIV/AIDS.

4. Nurses with HIV infection who are healthy should be treated the same as any other nurses. Nurses with HIV-related illness, including AIDS, should be treated the same as any other nurse with an illness.

5. The Code of Professional Conduct for the Nurse, Midwife and Health Visitor is a statement to the profession of the primacy of the patient's interest.

6. It is for this reason that the introductory paragraph of this code requires each registered nurse, midwife and health visitor to serve the interests of society, and above all to safeguard the interest of individual patients and clients. It is for the same reason that the Code goes on to indicate that each registered nurse, midwife and health visitor is accountable for his or her practice, and, in the exercise of professional accountability shall:

> act always in such a way as to promote and safeguard the well-being and interests of patients/clients
> ensure that no action or omission on his/her part or within his/her sphere of influence is detrimental to the condition or safety of patients/clients

7. It is the Policy of the Riverside Health Authority that members of staff who become HIV positive or develop AIDS shall retain their contractual rights of employment ('Members of Staff with HIV Infection' 10/05/88 Riverside Health Authority – Guidelines For Managers). The existence of HIV infection and illness due to the HIV infection, are not sufficient reasons in themselves for termination of employment.

8. Consequently, nursing personnel are encouraged to confide the nature of their HIV Anti-body status or illness to the Occupational Health Services. This will allow the nurse to be appropriately supported and cared for.

9. Nursing personnel who know they are HIV antibody positive or who have been diagnosed with an HIV-related condition must be under appropriate medical supervision. This can be their own Medical Practitioner or the Occupational Health Department. There is available within the Riverside Health Authority a comprehensive range of nationally recognised services and personnel with expertise in the care and support of individuals who are infected with HIV. Nursing personnel are encouraged to take advantage of these services and expertise which can be accessed through the Occupational Health Department.

10. Information regarding an employee's medical condition is confidential, as described in the Nursing Advisory Committee's previous Policy Statement on 'AIDS and Confidentiality' and Riverside Health Authority Guidelines ('Members of Staff with HIV Infection' 10/5/88). Information discosed to the Occupational Health Department is confidential. Positive counselling by the Occupational Health Department will encourage and support nurses in being able to share information with their line manager. If a nurse confides confidential information to their line manager, it may not be disclosed to other managerial colleagues without the express consent of the affected nurse.

11. The risk of HIV transmission from a nurse infected with this virus to a client is considered to be minimal. Currently, there is no known case where a client has become infected with HIV from contact with a Health Care Worker in an occupational setting. However, the small but possible risk which can exist, is described fully in Department of Health Guidelines ('AIDS: HIV-Infected Health Care Workers' March 1988). In most cases the risk can be eliminated by judicious use of gloves, waterproof dressings covering any open lesions and a high standard of personal hygiene (as per the previous NAC Statement 'Universal Precautions: HIV Disease' and current Infection Control Policies). All nurses employed by the Riverside Health Authority are required to comply with current control of infection procedures.

12. A theoretical risk may exist in nursing practice should an accidental injury to the nurse occur during a surgical invasive procedure where blood to tissue contact could occur. Clinical areas of particular concern may include the Operating Department, the Accident and Emergency Department and the Labour Wards.

Therefore, nurses known to be infected with HIV who perform or assist in such procedures must seek advice from the Occupational Health Department and their Manager. In each case, a careful assessment of the specific procedures undertaken by the nurse involved and the risk these may present to clients will be made. If a significant risk to clients is identified, then clinical re-assignment may be necessary.

13. Nursing personnel with HIV Disease may be susceptible to a wide range of illnesses which may affect their ability to work, including visual and mental impairment and/or infectious diseases. Clinical re-assignment of these personnel must be assessed by the Occupational Health Department and their Manager.

14. Nurses who are asymptomatically infected with HIV do not pose any special risk to clients of transmitting opportunistic or other non-HIV related infections. However, they should remain under regular medical supervision in order to ensure the early detection of infections, such as tuberculosis, measles and varicella. These can be contained by the same provisions that apply generally to infectious diseases affecting any nurse.

15. Nurses infected with HIV may be slightly more susceptible to infections such as tuberculosis, varicella or measles. The Occupational Health Department (in liaison with the Infection Control Officer/Consultant Microbiologist and the nurse's own physician) will be able to advise whether exclusion from contact with clients with these infections is necessary.

16. Reasonable and appropriate alternative clinical assignments will be made avilable to those nurses who require it as per numbers 12, 13 and 15 of this Policy Statement.

17. Screening facilities exist within the Riverside Health Authority for any member of staff who wishes to be tested for markers of HIV infection. The NAC has previously issued Policy Statements on both the requirement for true, informed consent for this test ('**AIDS: Consent For Serological Testing**') and the requirements for confidentiality in relation to the results of the test ('**AIDS and Confidentiality**'). These Policy Statements apply equally to the clients and the employees of the Riverside Health Authority.

18. Although there is no requirement for any employee to be screened for markers of HIV infection, we strongly advise that those nursing personnel who consider, on the basis of the known means of transmission, that they may have been infected with HIV, should seek immediate counselling and, if appropriate, diagnostic HIV anitbody testing.

19. Nurses affected or perceived to be affected by HIV/AIDS will be protected from stigmatization and discrimination by colleagues and clients. The Riverside Health Authority is committed to dealing effectively with all complaints of discrimination, victimization or harrassment.

20. The Riverside Health Authority is an equal opportunity employer and as such, has a legal obligation to ensure that the Authority itself, its employees and managers do not unlawfully discriminate.

21. Pre-emloyment HIV/AIDS screening is unnecessary and is not required. This refers to HIV antibody testing, assessment of risk behaviours and questions about HIV antibody tests already taken. However, potential nursing personnel employees who know they are HIV antibody positive are encouraged to confide in the Occupational Health Service. This will enable them to access the support and care available within the Authority and to obtain appropriate advice regarding clinical assignment.

22. The Riverside Health Authority is committed to offering the highest quality support and care to both its clients and employees and observance of these Guidelines promotes that commitment.

References:

Durman, L. (10 May 1988) **Memorandum to UGMs, District Directors: Guidance For Managers on Employment of Staff with HIV infection ('Members of Staff with HIV Infection')**, The Riverside Health Authority.

Expert Advisory Group on AIDS (March 1988) **AIDS: HIV-Infected Health Care Workers, Report of the recommendations of the Expert Advisory Group on AIDS**, Department of Health.

United Kingdom Central Council for Nursing, Midwifery and Health Visiting **(6 November 1989) UKCC Statement on AIDS and HIV Infection (PC/89/02).**

World Health Organisation (5 July 1988) **Consensus Statement: WHO Consultation on AIDS in the Workplace**, WHO Press.

World Health Organisation (1988) WHO AIDs Series 3, **Guidelines For Nursing Management of People Infected with Human Immunodeficiency Virus (HIV)**, p26, WHO in Collaboration with the International Council of Nurses, Geneva.

Department of Employment and the Health and Safety Executive (1987) **AIDS and Employment**.

Young, I. (31 December 1987) **Equal Opportunities Policy**, The Riverside Health Authority.

NAC (1987) **AIDS and Confidentiality**, The Riverside Health Authority.

NAC (1990) **Universal Precautions – HIV Disease**, The Riverside Health Authority.

NAC (1987) **AIDS: Consent for Serological Testing**, The Riverside Health Authority.

AIDS and cytomegalovirus

Previously, it was considered that as most patients with AIDS and AIDS-related illnesses were coincidentally excreting cytomegalovirus (CMV), pregnant health care workers should refrain from direct patient care activities with these patients because of the potential risk of CMV acquisition and possible subsequent damage to the developing foetus.

About 1% of women who lack CMV antibody become infected during their pregnancy. CMV can cross the placenta and infect the unborn child; in the UK about 3–4 per 1000 babies are born with CMV infection. Of those infected at birth, approximately 10–15% have an abnormality attributable to the virus.

Cytomegalovirus (CMV) is a common infection in the community. In the UK approximately 50% of women of childbearing age have CMV antibody which reflects persistent infection. Forty per cent of preschool children are found to be shedding CMV over a one year period and thus, pregnant women are frequently exposed to this infection.

Professor Catherine Peckham and Dr Don Jeffries prepared a report in August 1986 for the DHSS Advisory Committee on Dangerous Pathogens (ACDP) in which they concluded that 'although recent studies have shown that infection can be transmitted from young children to their parents, *there is no solid evidence that hospital nurses or nursery nurses are at increased risk of acquiring CMV infection from babies and young children or indeed any other patients in their care.*'

Their recommendations were:

There is no scientific reason why women of childbearing age or pregnant women should be excluded from contact with known excretors of CMV.

There is no indication for routine serological screening of female staff taking care of children or adults who may be excreting CMV because there is no evidence that CMV is an occupational hazard.

The most practical means whereby all women who are either pregnant or planning a pregnancy can be protected from acquiring CMV and other common infections in the community is by attention to good hygiene, for example handwashing.

The above measures suggested are consistent with those recommended in the US and Canada.

Therefore, *pregnancy in itself is not a contraindication for caring for patients who are or may be excreting cytomegalovirus (CMV).*

Index

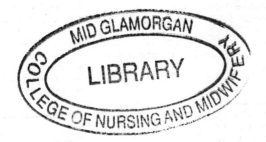